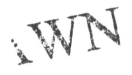

Ethical and Legal Issues in Home Health and Long-Term Care

Challenges and Solutions

Dennis A. Robbins, PhD, MPH
President
Integrated Decisions, Ethics, Alternatives, and Solutions
Westmont, Illinois
Former National Fund for Medical Education Fellow
Kennedy Interfaculty Program in Medical Ethics
Harvard University

AN ASPEN PUBLICATION®
Aspen Publishers, Inc.
Gaithersburg, Maryland
1996

Note: This book was prepared for readers who want to enhance the talent, tools, and techniques necessary for addressing a wide range of legal and ethical issues. Its goals are to provide helpful guidance and offer creative alternatives for dealing with challenges we face by equipping the reader with methods for identifying and addressing issues, defining alternatives, and therefore possibly preventing problems and conflicts from developing.

Before your organization decides to adopt the policies and techniques outlined in this text, it would be wise to enlist the services of a quality assurance representative, risk manager, and/or attorney. If conflict resolution is a matter of concern, it is vital that all discussions regarding the conflict be documented. Policies and procedures must be tailored to the specific organization, but also must be in accordance with state and federal law, practice acts, and other similar regulations. While the text offers suggestions and guidance for an attorney, it is not intended to provide legal advice or other professional counseling to the reader.

Library of Congress Cataloging-in-Publication Data

Robbins, Dennis A.
Ethical and legal issues in home health and long-term care:
challenges and solutions / Dennis A. Robbins.
p.   cm.
Includes bibliographical references and index.
ISBN 0-8342-0783-4
1. Long-term care of the sick—Moral and ethical aspects.
2. Long-term care of the sick—Law and legislation. 3. Home care services—Moral and ethical aspects. 4. Home care services—Law and legislation. 5. Life support systems— Moral and ethical aspects. 6. Life support systems—Law and legislation. I. Title.
RA973.R59   1996
174'.2—dc20
96-5377
CIP

Editorial Resources: Ruth Bloom
Library of Congress Catalog Card Number: 96-5377
ISBN: 0-8342-0783-4
Printed in the United States of America

1 2 3 4 5

To the three most important people in my life,
my daughters, Diana and Lynne,
and my wife, Lora

Table of Contents

Preface

This book is the result of ten years of working as a clinical ethics and health law consultant and teaching a wide variety of health care clinicians and executives. It addresses multifaceted legal and ethical issues in a way that is sufficiently comprehensive to account for their complexity.

Besides providing information on the development of legal and ethical issues in postacute care, this book focuses on the process of "doing ethics"—that is, the manner in which we approach and define issues, examine those issues, make provisional decisions, and test, revise, and justify those decisions. It is intended to be a resource for the reader who is unsure what to do when faced with a complex or overwhelming question. Guidelines that accommodate the reasonable and exclude the improper are a good starting point in the quest to make better decisions when faced with conflict, controversy, or uncertainty. Developing more dependable problem-definition and problem-solving skills can enhance our comfort in dealing with both legal and ethical issues, particularly those that arise in postacute care. The approach I've taken is to integrate a variety of perspectives to give a richer and more comprehensive treatment.

The models and alternatives I offer have been shown to be effective in teaching others to enhance their strengths and expertise and be able to resolve or preclude controversy and conflict when dealing with difficult issues.

I am frequently asked what training or education is required to be an ethics specialist in health care. That's a hard question. My background, for what it's worth, is as follows. After receiving a doctorate in philosophy (with advanced training in ethics) and teaching ethics for several years in a philosophy and religion department in the University of North Carolina system, I went back to school to pursue advanced work in medical ethics and health law. In the process I received an M.P.H. I was fortunate enough to be awarded a National Fund for Medical Education Fellowship for advanced study in medical ethics and health law through the Kennedy Interfaculty Program at Harvard, where I received my M.P.H.

During my fellowship, I served as a research fellow in medical ethics in the division of legal medicine and was an assistant in the Department of Geriatrics at Harvard Medical School. Upon completion of my formal education, I began teaching ethics and health law courses in graduate health administration programs and eventually assumed the directorship of one of those programs. At the same time, I began lecturing around the nation. I later left the directorship and became the chair of an institute on aging and subsequently worked full time as a clinical ethics and health law consultant, lecturing and consulting on ethical issues and policy development. For a period of three years I visited three or four different locations around the country each week. However, I missed the clinical exposure, so I began working as a clinical ethics consultant and became the director of a medical ethics service while maintaining a reasonably active but more moderate travel schedule.

The traveling I have done has allowed me to gain and maintain a national perspective and an awareness of emerging trends and innovative ideas. I have also worked with facilities to assess the viability and validity of their policies and procedures and bring them up to date on and help them incorporate the latest legal protections that could be afforded within the context of those policies. I offer special thanks to them, for without their energies and innovative spirit this book would not have been possible. They include Kerry Gillihan, then the CEO of Baptist Regional Medical Center (where the idea of an integrated policy was developed), Muhlenberg Regional Medical Center in New Jersey (the first facility to adopt an integrated policy), the Kentucky Hospital Association (the first state association to adopt the integrated policy concept as a guide for its member hospitals), and the Princeton Insurance Company (which featured programs on my integrated policy concept as part of its risk management program which aired nationally).

Being on the cutting edge in ethics and health law has been very rewarding for me. I have been able to keep current with new developments through working with such national organizations as the American Hospital Association, American College of Health Care Executives, American Medical Association, American Board of Utilization Review and Quality Assurance Physicians, American Health Care Association, American Association of Homes and Housing for the Aged, and several state-based organizations. My ongoing involvement in long-term and home health care and with hospitals and hospices has been an important source of knowledge as well. Working with attorneys, policymakers, state and national commissions, and regulators and judges has expanded my perspective and made me sensitive to the subtleties of the issues treated herein.

This book is intended to fulfill an unmet need in the home health care and long-term care literature. The contents are also applicable in hospice, community health, and other postacute settings. My objective was to cover a wide range of issues and topics, tools, techniques, and resources. Also, in my opinion, it makes little sense to discuss an ethical issue in home health or long-term care without first ensuring some understanding of what has happened to the patient at the acute care stage. My hope is that this book not only will be used as a resource but also can serve as a textbook for training and educating health care professionals. Accordingly, I have included an extensive bibliography.

The book is designed to help equip the reader to identify and address issues, define alternatives, and gain skills in solving and sometimes preventing problems and conflicts. When dealing with conflict resolution, it is particularly important to document the process of conflict resolution carefully and completely.

Before adopting the suggested policies and techniques in the book, you should tailor them to fit your organizational needs with the assistance of a quality assurance representative and/or risk manager and make sure that they are consistent with controlling state and federal laws and regulations. This book offers general guidance for your attorney, but it is not intended to provide legal or other specialized advice.

Acknowledgments

I would like to express gratitude to those who have enabled me to create this book. First, I would like to thank Ronald Scott Mangum, J.D., L.N.H.A., managing partner of Mangum Smietanka & Johnson, a health law firm in Chicago. His ideas on how to organize the book, his help on regulatory issues, and his advice on many legal matters were invaluable. I would also like to thank his legal and administrative office staff for their assistance in preparing and reviewing the manuscript.

I would like to thank Lora Robbins, Medical Librarian at Loyola Stritch School of Medicine in Maywood, Illinois, for developing the user-friendly bibliography. The time and energy she spent putting together such a helpful resource is greatly appreciated.

I am also grateful to those organizations, facilities, and individuals with whom I have worked as an advisor, consultant, educator, and problem solver.

Finally, I would like to reaffirm my thanks to the National Fund for Medical Education, which underwrote my postdoctoral studies in clinical ethics and health law at Harvard, and helped shape the intellectual and clinical foundation of this work. I also appreciate the helpful and supportive staff at Aspen Publishers, particularly Jane Garwood and Ruth Bloom.

1

Ethical and Legal Issues in Home Health and Long-Term Care: An Overview

Timely and clinically sensitive information with which to deal with ethical issues in home health care settings is virtually nonexistent, and issues in long-term care are just beginning to emerge. Although it is difficult to get accurate figures, there are over 21,000 long-term care facilities, 14,000 hospitals, and 38,000 nursing and personal care facilities.[1(p796)] Despite this vast array of institutional settings, some of the most interesting and challenging legal cases have arisen where the patient was no longer institutionalized and where caregivers were reluctant to make the same decisions as they might have made comfortably in a hospital or long-term care facility. Also, new Joint Commission on Accreditation of Healthcare Organizations (Joint Commission) guidelines call for health care organizations to address organizational as well as clinical ethical issues. These are likely to have dramatic implications for policy development and institutional mechanisms for conflict resolution.

It is difficult to obtain accurate and up-to-date guidance for addressing conflict, developing policies, and treating a wide range of ethical issues that generally arise in health care contexts. It is even more difficult to obtain guidance for addressing distinctive ethical issues in home health and long-term care. Obviously, since long-term care services can be provided in institutional settings, the community, and the home, the number of people receiving home care is uncertain, but it is estimated that almost three-quarters of the severely disabled who receive home care services receive that care from either family members or unpaid caregivers.[2(p5)] This in itself raises some interesting issues. For example, is appropriate or necessary care being provided and are health care professionals successfully identifying patient needs and filling in the gaps? This text was created to serve as a resource for creating, developing, and enhancing tools for identifying and addressing such issues and to provide workable solutions.

Growing controversy involving patients' wishes and rights, coupled with a growing demand for high-quality, effective care, has intensified the need for health care organizations to increase their capacity and to anticipate and address a wide spectrum of ethical issues as they arise. There are many forces shaping the development of ethical concerns in home health and long-term care and other sectors of postacute care. The more obvious forces include the trend toward managed care, new Joint Commission guidelines, regulatory issues, and increased fears surrounding legal liability. At the same time, there are new impetuses from within—a perceived need for some forum for developing and assessing policies and procedures for dealing with ethical issues, a need for educating the staff on current issues, and a need for some effective way of addressing ethical issues that arise internally or in an organization's relationship with other organizations across the health care continuum.

Home health care poses interesting legal and ethical issues partly because of the wide range of services provided as well as the different levels of acuity. Among the most obvious are high-tech home health issues, yet those with subtle and pervasive implications are often hardest to get a handle on. Long-term care issues are distinctive because of the extensive oversight and relative lack of independence that characterizes the long-term care industry.

Staffing issues, including the unavailability of services due to lack of staff who will advocate on behalf of the patient, have powerful implications for both long-term and home care. These issues are heightened partially because acuity is increasing in long-term settings and financial resources are uncertain.

The home care environment offers greater autonomy for both patients and caregivers. This autonomy can be a double-edged sword. It is helpful sometimes not to have someone always looking over one's shoulder, but occasionally it is essential to gain access to guidance and support, something not easy to do in a patient's home.

ETHICS AND BIOETHICS

There are some who prefer the term *bioethics* to *medical ethics* and the broader term *health care ethics*. *Bioethics* was coined in the late seventies when the field of medical ethics was begin-

ning to gain prominence in this country. One of the most interesting emerging issues in science and ethics at that time concerned recombinant DNA research and the possibility that
some aberrant strain would be let loose. Simultaneously,
medical ethics was expanding as a field in response to the
Quinlan decision. This case involved a young woman, Karen
Ann Quinlan, who had stopped breathing and was brought to
an emergency department and put on mechanical ventilation
to try to reverse her plight. The courts were being asked to
decide the question of whether or not life-prolonging medical
procedures should be withdrawn when the prognosis was
hopeless. The case was influential not only because of the legal
and ethical ramifications involved, and the role medical technology had in the decision-making process, but also the greatest question was who or what was to constitute the most appropriate forum for making such decisions? Bioethics
attempted to accommodate both types of issues; accordingly,
the term *bioethics* was coined.

Some critics of medical ethics in the United States have
claimed that only death-related issues are given a central, almost exclusive, place. Such critics have jocularly renamed bioethics as *biodeathics*. To avoid the implication that only end-of-
life issues are important and to avoid confusion with research
and science issues, the term *ethics* will be used in this book.
The range of topics, after all, includes professional issues as
well as issues concerning transfer and admission, continuity
of consent and care, access and availability, challenges posed
by managed care, unexamined opinions regarding how
changes in the way care is provided affect the ways in which
caregivers view patients, rationing, self-determination, high-
tech home health, death and dying, and several others.

LEGAL GUIDANCE INVOLVING END-OF-LIFE
   CONCERNS

No area of medical ethics and health law has received more
attention than issues that arise at the edges of life. Living wills
and other forms of advance directives have been touted as administrative and legislative panaceas. These, however, have
not settled the concern of caregivers, who struggle with personal and professional conflict under the cloud of perceived
legal liability. Serendipity often determines if a patient or resi-

dent is treated by caregivers who do not disenfranchise him or her or who enable decision making by the patient or his or her surrogate.

In the past 20 years, there have been a number of important legal cases that have provided guidance on how to deal with end-of-life decision making and the issue of informed consent. The first was the famous case involving Karen Ann Quinlan.[3] In this case, the court indicated that the duty to treat an individual diminishes as the individual's prognosis dims. Indeed, the court held that when the prognosis is one of hopelessness, the need to continue "extraordinary treatment" vanishes. It also stated that the legal involvement in end-of-life matters would "constitute a gratuitous encroachment upon the medical profession" and that such matters should be decided in a clinical forum.

The court case *Superintendent of Belchertown State School v. Saikewicz*[4] concerned the issue of substitution judgment. The court held that a surrogate decision maker, when acting on behalf of a decisionally incapacitated patient, must try to choose what the patient would have chosen had he or she been capable of making the decision. Further, the surrogate must try to take into account everything that would have had a material bearing on the patient's decision-making process.

The question of the legality of writing a DNR (do not resuscitate) order in advance of a health crisis was dealt with in the case *In re Dinnerstein*. The court held that this tactic was a reasonable extension of the substituted judgment standard and that such orders should be honored.

One of the most comprehensive attempts to provide guidance on how to approach end-of-life decisions by surrogates was undertaken by the court in the case *In re Spring*. The court actually set forth 13 different factors to be used in decision making by surrogates. Unfortunately the court did not tackle the question of what particular weight should be given to each factor, and so the court failed to clarify surrogate decision making to the degree it had intended.

In *Eichner v. Dillon*, the court stated that in end-of-life situations involving decisionally incompetent patients "any reasonable indication of patient intent will suffice." It rejected the alleged need for a cumbersome adversarial legal proceeding to determine whether life-prolonging medical treatment should be withdrawn or withheld.

Finally, the court in the case involving Nancy Cruzan tightened the standard of evidence to be used in surrogate decision making. This court held that the standard should be "clear and convincing evidence" of what the patient would likely have decided had he or she been competent to decide.

On the issue of honoring patient wishes, the legal legacy is confusing and contradictory. One thing that is clear is that the wishes of any patient should be ascertained as early in the treatment process as possible. Another is that the care providers should try to develop a sound knowledge of the legal and ethical concepts that apply to surrogate decision making, especially in end-of-life situations.

ETHICS AND POLICY DEVELOPMENT

In the past, providers often avoided dealing proactively with ethical issues.

> A recent study funded by the Robert Wood Johnson Foundation and reported by the American Medical Association as well as *The New York Times* . . . found wide gaps between what terminally ill patients wanted and what they got. Forty-nine percent of the patients who wanted to avoid cardiopulmonary resuscitation did not have DNR orders. The patients who did often had DNR orders written in the last two days; as a result half of these patients spent their last eight days either comatose or receiving mechanical ventilation in an intensive care unit. The second phase of study proved even more discouraging. Testing a system which was designed to help patients avoid unwanted life prolonging treatments by fostering better communication between patients and their doctors, the study found no change in ordering or the number of days that dying patients spent in undesirable states. Researchers involved in the study told *The New York Times* that every facet of medical culture, from the training of doctors to reimbursement systems to cover over reliance on high-tech treatment, conspired to cause doctors to ignore patients wishes. Most of us will die of an illness that will "not be labeled as dying until the last couple of days at best."[5] [(p5)]

Patients who were terminally ill or in the late stages of a degenerative disease, where interventions were likely only to prolong the dying process, were avoided because of unwarranted fears about legal liability. Much of the negativity surrounding end-of-life decision making can be defused if the necessary time and energy is taken to develop policies in advance of a crisis. Administrative policies can provide guidance for addressing ethical issues and also insulation against legal liability. They can increase the comfort level of caregivers and minimize discontinuity and mistakes, thereby reducing risk of a lawsuit.

Such policies should include

- a clear statement of the commitment of the health care organization to honor the wishes of patients
- guidance for clinical staff regarding documentation
- procedures for conflict resolution
- safeguards regarding patients' capacity to make medical decisions
- mechanisms to ensure continuity of patient consent

Well thought out policies create a framework for risk management activities. Investing energy in formulating policies is easily justified, and ultimately the energy required is less than the energy consumed in dealing with the uncertainties that exist in the absence of policies.

Policies should diminish recurrent problems so caregivers and administrators can deal with issues proactively rather than waiting until they get out of hand. While institutional settings vary, policies should offer guidance to clinicians and clarify the commitment of the administration to the community. Making policies available to patients can facilitate decision making and will show the organization cares about patient input and honoring patients' wishes. Good policies enable and support patients to make mature and informed decisions.

CONTINUITY OF CONSENT

Continuity across the health care continuum has particularly interesting implications for postacute care. In the case of continuity of consent, the goal is not only to identify patients' wishes from what they say and what can be gleaned from surrogates and family members but also to establish a foundation or database containing information about their wishes. Often during an extended hospital stay important information about decision making, the patient's wishes, and family dynamics is generated, information that could be extremely helpful for future decision making in other settings. It is important that there be knowledge of and access to this information. It is a serious omission, for example, to preclude information about the wishes of a long-term care resident who enters the hospital with an acute problem. The hospital should be supplied with pertinent information about the patient and the wishes and concerns that he or she voiced while in the long-term care facility. The transfer of such information helps ensure that the patient's wishes are honored, provides appropriate guidance, and increases the caregivers' comfort and confidence that they are doing the right thing.

The legal test in such circumstances is whether one exercised reasonable care. Showing that an extra effort was made to identify and act in accordance with the patient's wishes can often serve as low-cost legal protection. Caregivers can better serve patients and residents by ensuring that their decisions do not fall through the cracks when they are transferred from one health care setting to another. The increased flow of patients through the health care system has created added pressure to identify and communicate patients' wishes. Transfer policies should include

- procedures to identify and record patients' wishes
- procedures to ensure that the facility maintains information about current patients' wishes
- formal mechanisms to ensure that patients' wishes are transmitted from one health care setting to another

Continuity of consent has been made more complicated by the advent of managed care contracts, prospective reimbursement systems, and creative financing mechanisms. A patient's wishes documented during hospitalizations or treatment in other health care settings as well as the office records of the patient's primary care provider should be integrated into current and future decision making as a way of ensuring patient autonomy and addressing family conflict.

ETHICS COMMITTEES

There is increased pressure to create formal mechanisms for conflict resolution and policy development within health care. Ethics committees are increasingly being used as a means for dealing with ethical issues and resolving conflict of various sorts. They can also serve as a vehicle for mending the seams of the delivery system to ensure continuity of care and consent.

Institutional Ethics Committees

An institutional ethics committee specializing in home or long-term care deviates from ethics committees of the past. The first ethics committees to address long-term and home health care issues were offshoots of the committee in the Quinlan case, in which a potentially reversible acute episode occurred in an acute care setting on an emergency basis and it was suggested that a medical prognosis committee be created to assist in the decision-making process. This prognosis committee was referred to as an "ethics committee." This Quinlan model, however, was too restrictive to apply in most postacute care settings. This is not surprising, for the committee was a medical prognosis committee exclusively composed of physicians and was not equipped to handle many of the clinical and nonclinical issues that an ethics committee in home health, long-term, or other postacute care contexts needs to address.

Unlike the crisis management model found in many hospitals, a postacute care ethics committee should have an expansive role as a forum for the development of policies that affect patients' daily lives. Considerations when establishing an ethics committee include

- the type of committee and its membership
- the role, scope, and charge of the committee
- the use of consultants, clinical ethical tools, and clinical ethics rounds

The greatest opposition to ethics committees stems from clinical staff's concerns that these committees will question or interfere with staff decision making autonomy. One option for dealing with ethical issues, clinical ethics rounds, can provide an opportunity to address ongoing ethical issues for patients and staff as they occur. An ethics committee also can perform an "ethics audit" of decision-making guidelines to evaluate strengths and weaknesses as well as identify and respond to unmet needs in the organization.

Ethics Rounds

Ethics rounds can serve as an alternative for or a helpful supplement to an extant ethics program or ethics committee. They can also serve as a barometer for those facilities testing the possibility of creating an ethics committee for their facility or agency. Rounds are more often than not clinically based. They may be either separate ethics rounds or be included and integrated into existing patient care or specialized rounds. Rounds are well suited to clinical decision making as well as to solving or precluding emerging controversies. They can also serve as an interdisciplinary tool for challenging behaviors such as a physician who is reluctant to or delays in writing a DNR order. Rounds can be useful in terms of offering consistency in areas where inconsistency has been the rule rather than the exception in the past.

Community-Based Ethics Committees

A community-based ethics committee is intended to serve as a forum to meet many of the challenges associated with health care reform as well as respond to some of the pressures of managed care as patients travel across the health care continuum. A community-based committee can support continuity and consistency of care and consent across facility lines as well as deal with problems that require broader community integration and coordination than any one facility can provide. It should be part of an integrated community delivery and problem-solving system. It is a place where issues and problems can be addressed that individual facilities take neither ownership of nor responsibility for but that may dramatically affect the community. These include the problems associated with terminally ill patients who have indicated that they do not want to avail themselves of advanced cardiopulmonary resuscitation techniques. A community-based ethics committee also can address issues of continuity of effort, consent, and care between acute and postacute care settings as well as a wide range of community issues for which there is no other appropriate forum for identification and resolution.

TELEMEDICINE AND TELECARE

Telemedicine, including telehomecare, can increase access to health care. It can enhance health care providers' diagnostic capabilities by helping them to identify or rule out possible causes of illness. It can also aid them in supervising the provision of health care services to patients. For example, health professionals can use the phone to talk over case-related issues with family members ministering to the needs of a loved one in the home and can help create a support network between the patient and other patients. Telemedicine saves time and money and thus it can help fill in the gaps in care caused by tighter and tighter cost constraints.

It is essential, however, that telemedicine remains a supplement *to* and not become a substitute *for* hands-on care provided by trained professionals. In addition, there are obvious legal and ethical issues, including issues surrounding confidentiality, quality assurance, fraud and abuse, recordkeeping, and licensure, that need to be addressed by anyone who engages in this form of care provision.

ETHICS, MANAGED CARE, AND HEALTH CARE REFORM

Ethical issues in postacute care health care are arising increasingly because of challenges posed by integrated delivery and because of the shared risks and shared responsibilities of those who operate outside of the acute care setting. It is pointless to try to force an acute care model to deal with ethical issues in long-term or community health care. There are some fundamental differences that have to be acknowledged. The creation of integrated delivery systems makes it essential for each institution to know the strengths and goals of its partners in the delivery of health care and medical services.

Providers are increasingly required by regulators and state agencies to provide a certain level of care and at the same time are compelled by managed care contracts to provide that care at reduced costs. They are sometimes asked to limit care in situations in which they perceive patients to be at risk. As a consequence, they need to develop a framework for addressing such challenges and to create formal mechanisms to prevent patient care from being compromised. The problem is that they want the cadre of patients that a managed care contract offers but are afraid that deviations from the predetermined fixed ceiling will jeopardize the managed care contract, cause it to be withdrawn, or that they will be "de-selected."

Acute care settings are very different from postacute care settings. Whereas a hospital is a place to go to get well and then return home, long-term care often occurs in the home (or in a homelike environment) and can go on indefinitely. This creates the impression that long-term care is outside the continuum of care. The ethical issues are different as well, for long-term care is associated with legal and political problems from which hospital care, to some extent, remains insulated.

ETHICAL PRINCIPLES AND TECHNIQUES

Whatever course the future takes, there are some constants in the realm of professional duties and personal integrity. Caregivers must redirect their energies to develop a strong foundation to assess key issues. Resolving key issues in advance will reduce the agony of change. Caregivers need to ask basic questions, such as "Is the primary commitment as clinicians and administrators to those they serve?" At the same time, they need to readjust their thinking and focus on the question "What is right?" instead of "Who has rights?" They must also ask whether they are willing to compromise the way they provide care. Caregivers need to evaluate the roles and responsibilities to advocate on behalf of the patients.

Without policies and ways of enhancing one's capacity to deal with complex issues, ethics ultimately boils down to individual opinions. While opinions may have an important place in ethical discourse, they must be opinions that have been examined, tested, and revised and they must always be held provisionally and be open to further refinement. For this reason, ways of defining ethical issues and justifying and testing provisional decisions and will be covered later, as will a step-by-step model for addressing complex ethical issues (see Chapter 4).

ISSUES UNIQUE TO POSTACUTE CARE

Relationships with third parties are often especially challenging in both long-term care and home health. In fact, in long-term care there may actually be disincentives to act in accordance with patients' wishes caused by financial constraints and state regulations. To retain professional control, caregivers must anticipate ethical issues and address them in a knowledgeable manner. A community-based interdisciplinary ethics committee is one means of resisting pressure from managed care plans and state agencies. The primary ethical obligation of caregivers is to use their professional experience and talent to safeguard what is good and improve what is bad.

There are some issues that do not arise in all care settings. For example, a home care provider is invited into a home to provide needed care and support. The invitation is not without its perils, however. Independence and lack of oversight can sometimes breed unanticipated problems. One of these problems, which fortunately occurs rarely, is theft of the belongings of the person being cared for. In the home care setting, stealing is not as visible as in the acute care setting and may go on for a long period of time. In the hospital, it would be soon uncovered and the culprit would be fired. In the home care setting, stealing might even be intentionally overlooked if the family has had difficulty finding a caregiver. Family members may be convinced they would be left without any assistance in caring for their loved one.

Policies regarding ethical issues need to be assessed and be made consistent within and across departments, facilities, and even systems. These include policies on withholding or withdrawing life-prolonging medical procedures, conflict resolution, surrogate decision making, and a wide range of issues that arise in medical ethics and the ethics/health law interface. Educating staff about legal and ethical concepts is also a primary reason to establish an ethics program. Similarly, assessing in-house mechanisms for conflict resolution and creating an ethics committee or an ethics consultation mechanism can significantly improve the way ethical issues are addressed.

Many facilities are seeking advice and direction from existing ethics committees and are identifying helpful guidelines for dealing with ethical issues. They are also developing strategies for ethical analysis and better mechanisms to deal with ethical issues. Unfortunately, the integration of administrative and clinical ethics has not gone very far. However, renewed perspectives on patient and facility advocacy are now emerging, particularly in response to managed care.

EDUCATION AND POLICY DEVELOPMENT

A combination of policies, marketing, in-service education, and community education is the best avenue for turning the tide in this area. Clinicians need policies and support so they can be more clinically realistic and weave ethical decision making into the fabric of daily practice. Honoring patients' wishes and integrating them into the decision-making process seems easier than having to invoke the Constitution! It certainly is less cumbersome and costly than most legal proceedings.

Clear guiding policies can be particularly helpful when clinicians begin to learn to better cope with ethical issues and in so doing better insulate themselves against legal liability. The limbo time of uncertainty can be dramatically reduced, and the cost benefits become quite obvious in problem cases in which tens or even hundreds of thousands of dollars are at stake. Enhancing quality of care while making timely decisions can result in substantial cost savings.

A guiding policy can often give clinicians the approval they need to overcome a reluctance to proceed with or to discontinue a course of treatment. It enhances their confidence that they have satisfied their duty to act in accordance with professional standards and the wishes of the patient, and it maximizes liability protection by ensuring the existence of appropriate documentation.

In addition to supporting patient autonomy, allowing caregivers to perform without excessive fear, and allowing administrators to fulfill their commitment to those they serve, an ethics program can be an excellent marketing tool. An organization's communication of its willingness to honor the wishes of its patients will help attract people who are interested in getting high-quality care but do not want to become another Karen Ann Quinlan. By developing partnerships with patients and their families and gaining their trust, the caregivers can work with them and engage in joint decision making rather than usurp all patient care responsibilities or push them all onto family members.

Notes

REFERENCES

1. *Statistical Abstracts of the United States 1994: The National Data Book.* Washington, DC: US Department of Commerce Staff and Bureau of Census Staff, 1994.
2. Harwick S. *Across the States: Profile of Long Term Care Systems 1994.* Washington, DC: Public Policy Institute, American Association of Retired Persons, Center for Elderly People Living Alone, 1994.
3. *In re Quinlan*, 70 N.J. 10, 355 A.2d 647 (1976).
4. *Superintendent of Belchertown State School v. Saikowicz*, 370 N.E. 417 (1977).
5. New York: Project on Death in America. *Open Society Institute; PDIA Newsletter*. 1996, March; 1:1–8.

2

Internal and External Forces Leading to the Emergence of Ethical Issues in Home Health and Long-Term Care

THE DISTINCTIVENESS OF HOME CARE

The day I had set aside to rewrite this section started with my being given an insurance physical at home. While the electrocardiograph leads were being attached, my kitten, fascinated by the noise and the moving tape, attempted to attack the paper and pounce on the machine. The person operating the machine kept picking the kitten up and moving it out of the way, and the kitten, who assumed this was a new play partner, repeatedly vaulted back and forth on the machine, tried grabbing and clawing at the paper tape, and was entranced by the stringlike leads. Being hooked up to the leads, which were not adhering well, I called for my wife to help us out by removing the pesky kitten from the living room. She was busy and unable to assist. One of my daughters was away from home, and the other daughter, who was at home, was still sleeping. The home setting, usually so comfortable to be in, was creating some interesting and unexpected problems. This is a small example of the distinctive kind of difficulties that home caregiving is subject to.

The home must be modified to make it fit care needs without destroying the comfort and advantages of that setting, often a tough balancing act. In home health, because of payment constraints and the patient's homebound status, the patient often gets too little care for a protracted period of time. Nonprofessionals who fill in the gaps can hurt rather than help the patient, regardless of their good intentions. The professional caregivers must often coordinate inadequate support sometimes provided by persons incapable of doing assigned tasks. Identifying appropriate personnel and integrating clinical treatment and rehab requires more coordination than in the hospital, where everything is already there and all that is required to meet many needs is to make a request.

The desire to lay out the differences between home health and institutional-based care and the ethical and legal issues associated with these differences was an important motivation for my writing this book. Although the differences between long-term care and acute care are also noteworthy, I felt that it was essential to emphasize how dramatically dissimilar the home is to institutional settings, despite the fact that long-term care facilities take pride in their "homelike" atmosphere. In home health, someone is invited into the home and partially integrated into family life, something that does not typically occur in long-term care settings.

My intent in writing this book was not to minimize the seriousness of the ethical and legal issues that are common in acute care settings but to explore the ethical and legal issues that arise in postacute care in a way that takes into account their distinctiveness as well as their complexity. We all realize that the hospital of the recent past, of say, 25 years ago, is by no means the hospital of today and will certainly not be the hospital of the future. In the distant past, grandma could be left in the hospital for the weekend to "get a good checkup" while her kids went out of town. More recently, cost containment efforts and reductions in length of stay have provided strong incentives for early, earlier, and sometimes premature discharges. This has led to a greater focus on delivering health services and caring for patients outside of the hospital setting, a trend that will not only continue but be magnified. At the same time, every sector of postacute care is experiencing greater acuity and sicker patients. Accommodating these changes will require caregivers to revise how they view and approach problems and problem solving and to consider how to apply acute-care-level standards in the provision of postacute care.

Long-term care facilities and home health agencies must be prepared to anticipate and handle ethical issues as they arise. Several of the safeguards and protections that exist in hospitals are either diminished or lacking in postacute care settings, including quality assurance and risk management committees, morbidity and mortality conferences, numerous attending physicians, fellows and department heads, task forces, ad hoc committees, and CPR committees.

This is no great surprise. There are not enough health care professionals to staff many of these committees in home health and long-term care (although cross-institutional groups, such as community coordinating and community ethics committees, can perform some of these functions). Handling problems quickly and expediently is perceived to be more characteristic of acute care facilities. Yet it can be argued that many problems and needs are addressed effectively and efficiently in postacute care settings.

People often pride themselves upon using a certain hospital and will praise it loudly. Long-term care facilities are usually viewed as a "necessary evil," not a long-awaited place of residence. The home is an alternative to the sterility and medicalized environment of both the hospital and the long-term care facility. "High tech" home care medical technology is now being perceived as a means of keeping the home homelike and not medicalizing it to the point that it becomes barely distinguishable from an institutional setting.

THE DISTINCTIVENESS OF FACILITY-BASED LONG-TERM CARE

One distinctive problem in long-term care is that many emergency and medical procedures cannot be done in long-term care facilities, and so the patients sometimes need to be transferred to a hospital. This may take decision making out of their control. Hospitals have different perceptions, policies, and procedures than long-term care facilities, and the disparities manifest themselves quite clearly. If, for example, in an acute care setting caregivers need to determine that a patient is in a persistent vegetative state, they would make a stat neurological referral to rule out anoxic or ischemic encephalopathy. The examination would probably take place within 24 hours. By contrast, having a neurological exam in a long-term care facility may not be feasible, and the patient may have to be transported to a hospital. A home care patient would certainly have to go to a hospital, unless the patient has a good friend who is a neurologist, who has a relationship with the home care agency and who is willing to make a house call (which is *highly* unlikely). Not having medical information in a timely fashion, however, can delay decision making as well as cause additional anxiety for all involved. If sophisticated diagnostic equipment is needed and the patient must return to the hospital for a specific test, it becomes even more complicated and costly.

THE CHANGING ROLE OF HEALTH CARE PROFESSIONALS: RESPONDING TO THE PRESSURES OF MANAGED CARE

Managed care, particularly the kind of managed care where there is a capitated funding mechanism and certain designated benefits, can create an incentive to delay access to services. Strategies to contain or evade costs play a major role in many health care contexts. This has obvious implications for those who must have their medical needs met in a timely fashion. The lack of daily oversight on the part of medical providers may make this issue even more serious in postacute care settings. Acute care services demand more attention than other less dramatic kinds of interventions, and there are fewer resources available to challenge coverage decisions or limitations.

To better understand the various pressures created by imposing a marketplace model on health care delivery, it is necessary to unpack some of the covert issues associated with managed care. First, the insurer or payer of services under managed care is the driving force behind cost reduction. Unfortunately, the insurer often perceives both the patient and the health care provider as obstacles to maximize profit. The patient is perceived as a threat to profits, an overutilizer— someone who is fundamentally acquisitive and is willing to "game" the system to get as much as possible. The patient simply wants more, on this view, not necessarily what is best or most appropriate. Use is perceived as abuse, and hindering access to services is perceived as a legitimate protection against overuse. Patients no longer have the comfort of knowing that their needs will be appropriately met and that quality will not be sacrificed for cost. This is ethically problematic. While marginally beneficial services should be carefully evaluated, there should not be incentives to withhold or discourage or unreasonably delay appropriate care.

The rise of marketplace models of health care jeopardizes the distinctiveness of the individual patient. Capitated systems refer to the managed care patient as an "insured life." This is an unfortunate term. Nobody wants to be reduced to a number, yet being called an insured life implies an even *greater* reduction of individuality. It even has less distinctiveness than being called "the gallbladder in room 243" or "the guy in bed 2." Interestingly, patients are sometimes called "insureds" and perhaps that is all that is needed to satisfy shareholders. Life seems to have little or no meaning in this context. While this is an oversimplification, it does make an important point. A more generous approach might merely question the notion of a *capitated* system. *Capitation* derives from the Latin word *caput*, meaning "head," and the term suggests a "head count," again not a way of capturing individuality or the wholeness of a person. (*Capitation* is related to *decapitation*, which may bring to mind the question of whether the quality-cost interface is not a double-edged sword, as some think, but sometimes as impersonal as a guillotine in its cost-cutting mission.)

CHANGES IN PERCEPTIONS OF THE CAREGIVER-PATIENT RELATIONSHIP

There has been a great deal of reluctance to distance the patient from the caregiver-patient relationship by referring to the patient as something other than a patient (e.g., a client, an insured life, a covered life, an insured, a member, or a participant). In the caregiver-patient relationship, the patient puts him- or herself in the hands of the caregiver. The patient trusts that the caregiver has the knowledge and skill to help, heal, or advise the patient—to do what the patient cannot do on his or her own or to confirm that the patient has nothing to be concerned about. The patient relies on the caregiver's expertise and trusts that the caregiver will be forthright and professional in providing both information and medical services.

The caregiver-patient relationship is based on what the patient needs. Although the patient pays for services, when there is dire need or an emergency, care should be provided without concern for economic status or whether "911" should be called before the HMO. Even in the history of our fragmented American health care system, there have been provisions for offering care to those in need. This does not mean that the provisions have ever been adequate. The underinsured and uninsured still present a serious challenge to our health care system. Need has almost always overridden considerations of costs, but some changes now occurring in the health care setting are beginning to have dramatic implications for the way in which health care is perceived and are affecting (if not jeopardizing) the caregiver-patient relationship.

Perhaps a good way to explore these changes is to look at another professional field to see how clients are perceived there. Many people who work in the health care field have been reluctant to talk about their patients as clients. Clients are people who receive services in return for remuneration. In a lawyer-client relationship, noncompliance with advice or failure to pay is often the basis for dissolving the relationship. (Yet if a lawyer perceives that something needs to be done and the client has no ability to pay, the lawyer may choose work pro bono—without compensation.)

The question arises as to whether health care is simply a good or service to be sold on demand to a purchaser. The provider of clinical services–insured life relationship, as the caregiver-patient relationship might now be termed, has hidden implications that need to be unpacked. First, how does an insured life differ from a patient or a client? Second, if a doctor or any caregiver is no more than a supplier of clinical or specialty services, what implications does this have for current practice as well as the caregiver's historical role?

Even how we speak about care has changed. We have shifted from "utmost" care to the "highest-quality" care to "appropriate" care. Perhaps the next step will be to use a John Waynesque formulation—"Ya get what ya get and don't complain about it" care.

In addition, the physician has been transformed from a professional to a supplier of clinical services. Perhaps the next stage will be "retail clerk!" This demeaning reduction represents a dramatic departure from the physician's historical role. The physician is also viewed and evaluated as a profit center. Economic profiling of physicians includes identifying their utilization patterns. Data accumulated through profiling is often used to exclude or de-select physicians from participation in a given plan. As a result, caregivers are more sensitive to costs than they have been in the past. They also recognize the need to integrate the caveats of excess as well as what it means to be a professional into their decision-making patterns and processes.

There are two opposing views of human nature at stake here, the negative one already referred to (according to which patients and caregivers are profligate wasters of money and resources) and a more positive one. In the more positive view, the caregiver-patient relationship is based on trust and on a commitment to a common goal—the patient's health. The patient is a partner in the process of care, and the patient and caregiver jointly attempt to meet needs appropriately while minimizing unnecessary expenses so that the patient's premiums will not go up and the caregiver's profits will not decline. This model sets the stage for better care management, reduces duplication, and serves as a foundation for proactive rationing instead of thoughtless or serendipidous limit setting.

Having confidence that their needs will be met while knowing that some delays in access will occur (which is characteristic of managed care) may be something that patients will have to accept. Both caregivers and patients must try to balance the cost of proposed interventions against their efficacy in achieving desirable outcomes. Cost should simply be a factor to be reckoned with, not the driving force or mission. It is important that caregivers nurture a positive role for patients, because if they are only passive spectators, caregivers can expect a backlash of spiraling overutilization. It is also important that caregivers resist other people's attempts to redefine their roles and responsibilities.

It must never be forgotten that the patient is an important "asset." The patient can certainly be a financial asset. Without the dollars the patient or the patient's employer pays to the insurer, the insurer will cease to exist. If the patient is not treated as a partner in health care, the ability to effectively control costs through motivating healthy behaviors is lost. Caregivers need to think positively, not negatively, about those whom they serve. Strategic partnering should not be limited to institutions. Patients should be perceived as partners as well. The battleground can become a common ground.

The role of the caregiver and the role of the patient are facing unprecedented challenges. One fundamental question is, who is the customer—the patient or the plan? Pressures on physicians to weigh economy against need and to track costs and utilization as a condition of participation in a plan can be intense. Having to deal with incentives to reduce or restrict beneficial services is troubling, as are departures from the traditional doctor-patient relationship.

GATEKEEPING

Gatekeeping is a concept that is usually viewed negatively by patients and caregivers alike. It is seen as an impediment to access and availability, a hindrance that must be overcome. The physician or nurse who acts as the gatekeeper may appear to be merely a menial agent of the insurance company and not an advocate for the patient. However, historically the gatekeeper in fact has been an empowering agent, someone who gets the right thing done at the right time and who has an obvious and dramatic role in reducing inappropriate costs while putting no one at a disadvantage. The object of such a gatekeeper is not to ration care by making it difficult to access but rather to assist the patient by ensuring that appropriate services are delivered.

RATIONING

Another development which has dramatic ethical implications is rationing, which one author refers to as the R word.[1] Waste, medical futility, costs associated with the tactics of defensive medicine, ineffective treatment modalities, last-ditch efforts with minimal efficacy, exotic therapies, and reducing financial risks through lifetime caps are all topics being discussed more and more. Yet rationing remains a very confused concept, despite the fact that care is generally rationed, be it through nonreimbursement, restrictions on access or availability, gatekeeping, delays, or waiting lists. Rationing is either done covertly, which is more usual, or overtly. The goal of rationing is to rationally distribute something—to cut up the pie. Each person should have his or her own piece of the pie (ration), an amount that fulfills certain agreed expectations. The concept of unnecessary care arises when a person has already received his or her ration or is for some reason an inappropriate recipient of care. Of course, there is no need to consume one's portion of the pie if one is not hungry, particularly if the portion will be there if and when it is needed.

The topic of rationing has been repeatedly avoided in the American health care debate, while at the same time appropriateness is unquestionably tied to what is reimbursable and has been for some time. The failure to address this topic sensibly has resulted in a tourniquet approach to access to services and a failure to provide the American people with a consistent health care package and a sense of security.

There are many other less theoretical issues in managed care. Perhaps those that cause caregivers the greatest discomfort involve decisions that are clearly inconsistent with the way they practice or what they think is appropriate for the patient. In situations in which patients are vulnerable and in need of an advocate, caregivers' sense of ethical responsibility and fear of legal exposure blend.

There have also been attempts to publicly develop ways to allocate resources and set forth criteria determining what is appropriate and what is only marginally beneficial. The first statewide attempt to address such issues was the Oregon plan, which attempted to provide a much greater breadth of coverage for those in need than most traditional state Medicaid programs. The concept behind the Oregon plan was to extend coverage to those in need by openly discussing and prioritizing the allocation of resources to meet the needs of a wider spectrum of people. The goal was to reduce the use of marginally beneficial services and ensure the use of effective ones. What is interesting about the Oregon plan is that allocation issues were addressed in a publicly observable forum and were not left to be decided through chance.

Factors such as efficacy, benefit to the individual, benefit to society, the meeting of unmet needs, and the like, are integrated into the Oregon plan. It appears that there is minimal quibbling about whether a person will get services so long as the person's condition is listed as covered. The plan is intended to give greater access to a greater number of people rather than provide only emergency services for a select few and a wide range of services for others who are Medicaid eligible. This approach tries to offer equity for a large group of citizens and is a laudatory attempt at fairness and access.

IMPLICATIONS OF CHANGES IN HEALTH CARE PARADIGMS

If the roles of patient, provider, and payer in the health care system do not change for the better, we run the risk of devolving further into distrust and dislocation. There is no stronger reason to try to provide an ethical underpinning for today's health care debate than the chaos in which we are currently enmeshed. Ethics will not by itself solve the health care dilemma, but it offers a reasoned approach, based on traditional American values, to the evaluation of possible solutions.

As already discussed, managed care, particularly capitated systems, has caused drastic changes in the way that patients and providers are viewed. It also poses distinct ethical dilemmas for both patients and providers. Providers are being forced to integrate their operations with and subject their caregiving procedures to the scrutiny of managed care organizations.

Health care traditionally has been an area in which collaboration and sharing, for some, were standard. This paradigm has shifted, however, and now for some, the primary concern has become cost. Hidden amidst the focus on cost and efficiency are presumptions about the role of the caregiver and the patient. The caregiver-patient relationship—one of intimacy and shared trust—is being replaced by a supplier of clinical services/insured life relationship. Transforming the caregiver into a mere supplier of services shifts the caregiver's role from compassionate teacher to functional agent whose job is to control costs for the payer. In that role, how do health care professionals maintain the autonomy necessary to perform their traditional mission of caring?

LEGAL RESPONSES TO COVERAGE DECISION CONTROVERSIES

Wickline v. State of California

The ethics of caregiving requires that providers give to their patients the care necessary for the patients to heal. Doctors are bound by the Hippocratic Oath to do that which is within their power to assist patients and are proscribed from taking actions that will harm patients. What happens when a caregiver believes that a procedure is medically necessary for the patient to heal but the managed care organization refuses to authorize the procedure? First let us unpack some of the presumptions operant here. The "refusal to authorize" is a standard euphemism for "refusal to pay." But the caregiver is still obligated to provide medically necessary procedures. This situation was addressed by the California Supreme Court in 1986 in *Wickline v. State of California*.[2]

In *Wickline*, the patient entered the hospital with a venous insufficiency in one leg. The insufficiency was caused by a constriction of a major blood vessel in the lower back, and the accepted treatment was to surgically graft a new section of blood vessel into the back. After the surgery, Mrs. Wickline's attending physician ordered her to remain in the hospital for eight days. Mrs. Wickline was a beneficiary under the California Public-Aid-system, Medi-Cal, which required pre-authorization for a hospital stay of that length. The Medi-Cal reviewer denied coverage for an eight-day stay but did allow Mrs. Wickline to remain in the hospital for four days. Her attending physician felt that it was useless to make further attempts with Medi-Cal, and at the end of four days Mrs. Wickline appeared to be stable and was discharged to her home. Several days later, she was readmitted with advanced gangrene due to failure of the graft to heal properly. Her leg was amputated and she sued Medi-Cal.

The court examined the circumstances and felt that, while a third-party payer such as Medi-Cal could be liable for negligently implementing a medical cost containment system, it was the physician who bore the brunt of responsibility for appropriate care. The physician could and should have been a stronger advocate for his patient, with the consequence that Mrs. Wickline's leg might have been saved. The case was remanded to the lower court and presumably settled, because there is no further legal disposition. *Wickline* established that a third-party payer may be liable under some circumstances, although what these circumstances are remained an open question. Clearly, the physician is always an independent intervening agent, and so only when the physician has exhausted all remedies, including, probably, the delivery of uncompensated care, and continued care would necessitate payment by the third-party payer, will the payer be liable. The courts will *first* look to the professional health care provider to assess liability for negligent treatment. As recently as March 1996, a case was brought against a nurse and a home health agency alledging that the failure to refer resulted in the amputation of the patient's leg.[3]

Other Cases

A recent article in *The New York Times* dealt with legal responses to coverage decisions on the part of insurers for advanced medical treatment.[4] Needed care that may have been specifically excluded in an insurer's policy was the focus. Within the past five years there has been a "dramatic increase in lawsuits provoked by insurance industry denials for medically advanced treatment."[4] The article indicated that even when Employee's Retirement Income Security Act (ERISA) may obligate a court to give the benefit of doubt to the insurance carrier, patients have nevertheless been successful in their challenges by "demonstrating that the treatment they need is sufficiently advanced and accepted to warrant coverage."[4] Ten states have already passed some versions of legislation mandating that coverage be available for new treatments that have been demonstrated to be accepted by the health care profession.

Even without the concern of legal liability, various state regulatory schemes require certain levels of health care services to be made available to all patients. Yet most managed care plan contracts fail to recognize that any regulatory or professional body outside of the plans' own medical reviewers can determine what care is appropriate. A recent lawsuit (*Fox v. Healthnet*)[5] of $89.3 million has been settled for an undisclosed amount based on the failure to inform a patient of the results of a test that would have resulted in costly treatment. Other large awards have been provided, as well as lifting of the gag rule which resulted in several lawsuits. The gag rule had previously precluded the communication of treatment options if they were not covered services within a specific plan.

The conflict between clinical judgment and cost containment cannot be resolved easily. Providers can only be expected to give so much uncompensated care. The problem is exacerbated by foreigners in dire need of medical care who come into the United States seeking uncompensated services, an issue that has to be addressed with both delicacy and fairness.

So how can the problem be resolved? A firm ethical foundation for determining at what point caregivers can no longer be expected to deliver free care will provide a strong defense against legal and ethical challenges. Certainly, developing such a foundation is preferable to pushing the problem aside, particularly when it may seriously threaten the continued viability of the facility or agency for which the caregivers work.

Managed care will continue to challenge the ethical limits of professional health care until providers, patients, and payers can be viewed as partners in the delivery of appropriate health care. Until then, providers need to be given back their role as advocates and protectors of patients.

AMA Guidelines

The AMA has created some guidelines to deal both with the *Wickline*, *Fox*, and related cases, and other legal responses to coverage decisions including the $89 million Fox award referred to. Some of their key elements are listed below:[6]

1. The duty of patient advocacy is a fundamental element of the physician-patient relationship that should not be altered by the system of health care in which physicians practice. Physicians must continue to place the interests of their patients first.

2. When managed care plans place restrictions upon care that physicians in the plan may provide to their patients, the following principles should be followed:

   (a) Any broad allocation guidelines that restrict care or choices—which go beyond the cost benefit judgments made by physicians as part of their broad professional responsibilities—should be established at a policymaker level so that individual physicians are not asked to engage in ad hoc bedside rationing.

   (b) Regardless of any allocation guidelines or gatekeeper directives, physicians must advocate for any care they believe will materially benefit their patients.

   (d) Adequate appellate mechanisms for both patients and physicians should be in place to address disputes regarding medically necessary care. . . . The physician's duty as patient advocate requires that the physician challenge the denial and argue for the provision of treatment in the specific case. Cases may also arise in which a health plan has an allocation guideline that is generally unfair in its operation. In such case the physician's duty requires not only a challenge to any denials of treatments. . . but also advocacy on the health plan's policymaking level to seek an elimination or modification of the guideline. Physicians should assist patients to seek appropriate care outside of the plan when the physician believes the care is in the patient's best interests.

(f) . . . the physician's obligation to disclose treatment alternatives is not altered by any limitations in the coverage provided by the patients' managed care plan. Full disclosure includes informing patients of all their treatment options, even those that may not be covered under the terms of the managed care plan. . . .

(g) Physicians should not participate in any plan that encourages or requires care at below minimum professional standards.

REGULATORY ISSUES

The Patient Self-Determination Act

Perhaps the primary regulatory initiative that has heightened recent awareness of ethical issues in health care is the Patient Self-Determination Act. This act, which became effective December 1, 1991, requires that all health care providers who participate in the Medicare or Medicaid programs inform their patients, prior to providing health care services, of their right under state law to make an advance directive. While this law would seem to arise from the caring concern of a government interested in protecting patient rights, the act originated as part of an attempt by the Health Care Financing Administration to reduce the number of costly Medicare and Medicaid outliers who were consuming an undue portion of health care funding, including patients in a persistent vegetative state on artificially supplied life-supports. Although the original motivation for the act was cost containment, most health care providers have agonized over the rights and responsibilities of patients and providers in end-of-life decision making.

On its face, the act is easily complied with. The provider makes a perfunctory inquiry as to whether the patient has an advance directive, charts the answer, and hands the patient a sheet of paper that summarizes state law on advance directives. From a records review perspective, the act's mandates have been met. In actuality, providers do attempt to behave in accordance with the spirit of the act, but they often misunderstand their legal and ethical options. Patients may request unclear and ambiguous directives such as "no heroic measures" and "do not resuscitate" orders with little understanding of the clinical situations in which such orders are appropriate. Physicians, afraid of legal liability, fail to adequately inform patients about their options and then fail to carry out the patients' wishes through appropriately written medical orders.

In some cases, providers actually have disincentives to follow the act. Home health and long-term care providers are reimbursed based on the number of days or times that they provide services to patients. Servicing a patient in a persistent vegetative state might mean a healthy "annuity" for a provider. In addition, regulators seem to expect unrealistically high results from health care delivered to the elderly population. The last few months of life are medically the most expensive. In this period, people become increasingly frail, ill, and then die. Regulators as well as many well-intentioned providers would like to reverse the dying process. Some see death as a failure of care, so permitting a patient to die without taking all possible measures to sustain some type of sentient existence appears unacceptable. In fact, the regulatory process of patient assessment and care planning to assist patients to attain their "highest practicable" functioning encourages providers to try to achieve unrealistic results, and early death as a result of a properly executed and followed advance directive becomes hard to deal with emotionally. The aforementioned Robert Wood Johnson study noted that even with advanced training in developing better communication skills, there was "no change in DNR ordering or the number of days that dying patients spent in undisirable states."[7]

Medicare and Medicaid Fraud and Abuse

In 1977, the Medicare and Medicaid acts were amended to prohibit any type of payment or consideration for referrals of Medicare and Medicaid beneficiaries. In its simplest form, the law is easy to understand. It is illegal to pay or provide consideration to anyone as a lure for referral of patients for health care services covered by Medicare or Medicaid. Unfortunately, interpretation of the law has become much more complex. The issue of consideration has expanded from the simple payment of money to include any type of benefit provided at less than full market value. For example, a pharmacy may provide a computer terminal to a hospital or nursing home so it can electronically order drugs and medicine for patients, or a medical equipment supplier may provide training to facility staff designed to ensure they know when to order and how to use supplies. In both cases, the benefits have traditionally been provided to the health care providers free of charge. Such practices have been curtailed or discontinued because of court decisions that have held that if *any* part of the intent of providing a benefit is to encourage referrals, the entire transaction is poisoned.

The ethical and legal problem is to be able to determine which relationships *inappropriately* taint a health care provider's clinical judgment. Because of the almost unlimited variations on this theme, a provider who blithely ignores referral issues runs a substantial risk of severe penalties, including, very likely, exclusion from any participation in the Medicare or Medicaid programs for a minimum of five years. This is a penalty that would bankrupt most providers. Showing that a relationship in which some benefit is provided at less than full market value is ethically correct and justified by the health care mission of the provider can be critical to defending against a fraud or abuse charge successfully.

Stark Antireferral Regulations

Another initiative that seems ethically motivated but is really intended to reduce health care cost is the physician antireferral legislation sponsored by Representative Pete Stark. The original legislation, part of the Omnibus Budget Reconciliation Act of 1989, refused Medicare and Medicaid payment for any service rendered by a clinical laboratory that was referred to the lab by a physician who had a financial interest in the lab. This law was prompted by a study conducted in Florida that showed massive overutilization of lab services by physicians with a financial interest in the labs they referred to. Effective January 1, 1995, the prohibition was expanded to cover additional designated services.

Although compliance with the self-referral laws and regulations primarily depends on their interpretation, there are so many different types of relationships between providers and physicians that some mechanism is needed to sort out which are necessary for the delivery of appropriate health care services. Relationships in this category can be defended against most legal attacks, while those that are not will pose a risk of severe penalty.

Regulatory challenges can only be successfully dealt with by a thorough understanding of the legal and ethical ramifications of appropriate delivery of health care services. The issues are often framed in terms of legal liability, but because of the inexact and changing nature of the laws dealing with end-of-life decisions, provider relationships, and other "legal" issues, virtually every such legal issue involves ethical precepts.

JOINT COMMISSION ON ACCREDITATION OF HEALTHCARE ORGANIZATIONS MANDATES

The Joint Commission on Accreditation of Healthcare Organizations is a private body that accredits various types of health care providers according to standards developed by it. The Joint Commission was formed by the American Medical Association, the American Hospital Association, the American College of Surgeons, and the American College of Physicians. Other than the privately recognized prestige of its accreditation, the Joint Commission would have little relevance to providers but for the prevalence of Medicare reimbursement. Several years ago the federal government made a determination that accreditation by the Joint Commission was equivalent to certification that a hospital or nursing home complies with Medicare conditions of participation. More recently, Joint Commission accreditation was extended to home health agencies and can be expected to be extended to other types of health care organizations in the future.

So Joint Commission accreditation provides automatic Medicare certification. So what? Many believe that annual Medicare surveys are true bureaucratic compliance inspections. The surveyors, who are salaried government employees, may not give assistance, and in many ways the success of the survey system is measured by how many deficiencies are discovered and how many providers are denied Medicare participation. Joint Commission surveys, on the other hand, are conducted by peer professionals who actively practice in the field. The surveyors provide observations and recommendations to the providers to assist them in achieving compliance with the standards. They are "gentler, kinder" evaluations, and success is measured more by the number of providers who are helped to achieve higher standards than by the number found to be deficient. Once accredited by the Joint Commission, a provider may be deemed in compliance with Medicare standards for up to three years and can use the interim period to improve patient care rather than frenetically prepare for its next Medicare survey.

The Joint Commission has had clinical ethics standards for years. These standards require health care providers to have mechanisms in place to deal with clinical issues and maintain a high level of quality. The Joint Commission has expanded its ethics standards to include "organizational ethics." The intent of these standards is to encourage providers to address issues of access to and availability of services, resource allocation, and interorganizational referral and payment systems. That they have been added on is a reflection of the reality of managed care and the shrinking public tolerance for rising health care costs. Their addition is also a response to legislative initiatives to reduce inappropriate utilization of health care resources, such as the anti-referral laws sponsored by Representative Stark. By causing providers to deal with the ethical implications of inappropriate referral and utilization pressures, the Joint Commission hopes to reduce the need for further legislative and regulatory restrictions in this area.

Even for providers who are not Joint Commission accredited and have no intention of becoming so accredited, Joint Commission standards are important because they are often used as models for federal and other third-party regulatory and payment standards. What is a Joint Commission recommendation today will likely become a federal regulation tomorrow.

LEGAL LIABILITY

Fear of Legal Liability

The easiest way to strike fear into the hearts of most health care professionals is to threaten to sue them. Frequent publicity about multi-million-dollar jury verdicts reminds health care professionals that a misstep can be incredibly costly. The concern over whether an action is right or wrong is dwarfed by the worry that the time and expense involved in defending a lawsuit, not to mention the adverse publicity, will simply be overwhelming. Fortunately, the publicity belies the facts. As often as not, health care professionals are exonerated in court, and in some cases reverse suits against careless plaintiffs for abusing the legal system or suing frivolously have paid off. But it is the perceived risk of legal liability that can drive a cautious health care provider to practice inappropriately.

Only in a perfect world could the claim be made that every law protects right action. Laws are imperfectly written to correct imperfectly perceived situations. As a result, what would appear to the mythical "reasonable person" to be proper is often in fact illegal. So what does ethics have to do with protecting against legal liability? It is generally acknowledged that if the party to a lawsuit can demonstrate he or she pursued a logical and ethically based approach, he or she is likely to either succeed in litigation or to minimize his or her liability. The ability to frame ethical and legal issues and to use ethical principles to justify an action can be critical to success.

The ethical pressures listed above would be difficult enough to deal with in a cooperative society. Add to these the real or perceived exposure of health care providers to legal liability and the situation becomes explosive. Many fears of legal liability are based on a misunderstanding of the legal concepts involved in duty, negligence, and injury. An understanding of these concepts not only reduces fear but permits the planning of protective clinical and organizational measures. Clearly, informed legal counsel is critical, but just as critical are informed clinicians. Likewise, decisions based on a thorough prior examination of the relevant issues will usually be respected by a court reviewing provider actions months or years later. If the provider response to a crisis, although not perfect, is rational and carried out in accordance with carefully crafted policies, much legal protection will be afforded.

The concern with legal liability arises more from misperception than from reality. In the following chapters, recommendations on how to insulate oneself against legal liability are included. The recommendations pertain to, among other topics, ethics committees, clinical ethics rounds, informed consent, patient rights, documentation, and, especially, the development of policies and procedures.

Negligence and Malpractice

In this section, a short excursion into the concepts of negligence and malpractice is provided. *Malpractice* means bad practice. The expectation is that there be good practice. Since it is perceived that people have a right to good practice and its results, when they get bad practice and the accompanying bad results, they may choose to seek compensation for the loss or injuries they suffered.

In any negligence claim, someone is alleged to have failed to provide something—good practice. Most negligence in health care also involves consent, specifically informed consent. A patient consents to a procedure but the expected results do not occur.

The field of tort law deals extensively with questions of duty and negligence. Negligence includes everything from leaving a surgical instrument in a patient to performing the wrong procedure, doing surgery on the wrong patient, or allowing a serious complication to occur because of lack of follow-up, or failure to make a timely and appropriate referral.

The following framework can often be helpful in assessing potential liability. There are four components that must be present if an allegation that negligence occurred is to be worthy:

1. *A duty owed.* Did someone have a responsibility to do a certain thing in a certain way? If not, there was no duty; if so, there was a duty.

2. *A breach of duty.* If it has been established there was an affirmative duty, the question arises whether there was a failure to fulfill or act in accordance with that duty.

Even if there was an affirmative duty but there was no breach of that duty, negligence cannot be demonstrated.

3. *An injury.* The patient must have suffered an injury or related damage as a result of the breach of the duty owed.

4. *A proximate cause. Proximate* means very near, and a proximate cause is an event or action directly causally related to the injury that occurred. If the caregiver's breach of duty (failure to perform or act in a certain way) was causally related to the patient's injury, there is a high likelihood that a legal action could successfully be brought.

In cases involving strict liability, one might not have to show fault but only show that something occurred. Sometimes the principle of *res ipsa loquitur* (the thing speaks for itself) comes into play. For example, if a surgical sponge is left inside an individual, that sponge, strange as it may sound, speaks for itself; it would not be there unless someone involved in the surgery had left it there. The patient had no control over the placement of the sponge. If a medical device or pharmaceutical, after being offered to a patient with the assurance that the product is safe, is later discovered to cause injury or death, strict liability can be demonstrated solely by the fact that the product was used and the patient has an injury (examples are the recent challenges against the tobacco industry).

CASE STUDIES

Case 1

A home health nurse and a live-in nurse's aide are taking care of a patient who has sufficient income to afford their full-time help. The patient is borderline in terms of capacity.

The nurse has overheard the aide asking the patient for money and sharing hard luck stories. The patient is good-hearted and tears fill her eyes. She is also afraid that if she doesn't financially help the aide, she will lose the support she so desperately needs. As a result, she gives money to the aide frequently as well as unlimited access to her checkbook.

One day the nurse is asked to help the patient write a check to pay for a delivery of some Chinese food. She observes in the checkbook that every week at least $200 is being paid for groceries. Yet she knows there is never much food in the refrigerator—some juice, some eggs, and maybe a package of ground beef. Perhaps the aide is taking the food home. Also the issue of substantial amounts of money being given away to a caregiver above and beyond their professional fees for their services for anyone but particularly for someone vulnerable and at risk is another issue. So many people who are older and living at home and requiring supports, living on a fixed amount of money from Social Security and some inheritance, may feel that they have to buy their caregiver's allegiance in this way. Accepting such sums from someone who probably does not realize what's going on is wrong for the caregiver. The nurse also notices a loose switchplate cover and goes into the basement to get a screwdriver to tighten the loose screw. She finds that all the tools are also missing. The last time she saw them was two days ago, when the aide's boyfriend was in the house doing repairs. (She also determined from looking at the checkbook that the charge for the repairs was much higher than was reasonable.)

- What should the nurse do?
- Does she have a responsibility to try to protect the property assets of the patient?
- What legal issues are involved should the nurse fail to act?
- Does the home care agency have a duty to identify the problem?

Case 2

A large university-based practice known for its innovativeness and its high-quality services gets a large percentage of its business from managed care. The managed care insurers have been rather slow to respond to innovations even when they are less costly and more effective. An HMO patient requires a procedure performed. One of the surgeons has been

using a new technique for her patients that is safer, less trau-
matic to the tissue, faster, and more effective; creates less morbidity; and is less costly to perform. However, the patient's
HMO will not authorize the new procedure.

- What is the problem, if any, with using the new technique?
- What responsibility does the surgeon have?
- What responsibility does the administrative director of the
  practice have?
- What role might the patient or his surrogate play in this
  matter?
- What role, if any, might the courts play in this matter?
- What legal issues are involved?
- Does the surgeon's action constitute fraud and what ex-
  actly does that mean?

Case 3

A case manager has requested a service for a patient who
does not quite meet the eligibility criteria for that service. She
has learned that creative writing is one means of getting care for
borderline patients—those not quite sick enough to be okayed
for services by the insurer. This tactic and others like it have
become standard practice, and the case manager feels justified
in using them because she is convinced they help her ensure
that her patients get the care they need.

- Is anything wrong with her actions?
- To whom does she have a responsibility?
- Should lying be a precondition of care?
- How does this fit in with the mission or organizational eth-
  ics guidelines of the agency or company?

REFERENCES

1. Havighurst C. Prospective self-denial: can consumers contract today to
   accept health rationing tomorrow? *University of Pennsylvania Law Review.* 1992;140:1755–1808.
2. *Wickline v. State of California*, 239 Cal. Rptr. 805, 741 P.2d 613 (1987).

Notes

3. Suit filed in Circuit Court, March 1996, Baltimore, Maryland of a Severna Park registered nurse and Staff Builders Home Healthcare of Baltimore. Reported in Capital Gazette Communications Newsletter, March 13, 1996.

4. Gallinari K. Relieving insurance pain for patients and courts. *The New York Times*. November 5, 1995.

5. *Fox v. Healthnet,* ND #219692, Cal. Super. Ct. Riverside Cty (December 1993). Settled January 1994.

6. The Council on Ethical Affairs of the AMA. Ethical issues in managed care. *Journal of the American Medical Association*. 1995; 23 (4):330–335.

7. New York: Project on Death in America. *Open Society Institute, PDIA Newsletter*. 1996, March; 1:1–8.

3

Foundations and Applications in Ethics: Understanding Principles for Addressing Ethical Issues

THE PROCESS OF DOING ETHICS

Ethics, Morals, and Ethical Theory

There is frequent confusion among health care professionals as to what ethics really is. They tend to think ethics includes any difficult question that is not easily squeezed into some etiologic framework or established procedure or protocol. How they deal with ethical questions is even more disturbing. Many are of the opinion that they merely have to raise a question and show how really difficult it is. Having done this, they seem to think they can either ignore it or use its complexity as an excuse for not dealing with it. Articulating or raising a question is not equivalent to addressing it. If one really wants to address ethical questions seriously, there must be some rationale for constructing and evaluating principles and then providing a basis for justification of their rationale. This involves examining the principles carefully, weighing alternatives, and deciding what principles most appropriately address the issue at hand.

Ethics is a field of study that deals with concepts and principles surrounding what is right and wrong (and good and bad) and how we justify our assertions and judgments about right and wrong. Ethics and morals are often viewed as exactly equivalent. This is not correct. Ethics deals with principles of right and wrong and justifications of ethical judgments, whereas morals deals more with how we apply these principles and judgments to our daily behavior. Morals is tied to sentiments—how we "feel" about something. Ethics is aligned more closely with principles and "reason."

Historically, the distinction between ethics and morals can be traced to the seventeenth century, when the opposing theories of rationalism and empiricism were fighting it out on the field of honor. Rationalism is a theory of knowledge that asserts we gain knowledge primarily through reason. The best-known proponent of rationalism, Rene Descartes, even went so far as to write a detailed treatise called *Rules for the Direction of the Mind*. On the other hand, the empiricists felt that we gain knowledge primarily through the senses. David Hume, a proponent of empiricism, believed that an idea or rational construct is weak when compared with an original feeling. Remembering you burned your hand and actually burning it, he argued, are vividly distinguishable.

Ethics and its principles are more closely associated with the rationalist tradition, and morals more with sentiments (how we feel about something and why we feel the way we do). It is important to recognize this distinction. In this book, the focus is primarily on principles and concepts and the way in which we justify them. In other words, the focus is on ethics. (This fact should not be taken as an indication that morals are not important.)

Consequentionalism and Nonconsequentionalism

Many feel overwhelmed by the intricacies of ethical theories and ultimately believe that ethics boils down to individual opinions. Such people make little distinction between *examined* opinions that have been carefully tested and *unexamined* opinions. To minimize the feeling of being overwhelmed, it is essential to understand the difference between consequentionalism and nonconsequentionalism. If you serve or will serve on an ethics committee or merely want to sharpen your own skills and tools for clarifying and resolving issues, knowing the difference will enhance your confidence and comfort. It will allow you to be clearer about how people justify their opinions and to what type of justification they appeal.

Consequentionalism and nonconsequentionalism are broad categories that encompass many different ethical theories. Consequentionalism asserts that the rightness or wrongness of a given course of action or choice is determined primarily, if not exclusively, by its consequences or ends. This may bring to mind the well-known but controversial principle that "the end justifies the means." Those who have heard this principle may wonder whether consequentionalism is able to take into account the depth and complexity of most ethical issues. In actuality, consequentionalism is a very helpful way of critically evaluating or justifying such issues. A person using a consequentionalist theory will attempt to assess an array of possible results of different courses of action. Then, based on the probability of the different results and their degree of goodness, the person will identify the best course of action. Also, testing provisional theories and judging them in the light of possible counterexamples is a way of determining the best or most appropriate alternative.

Nonconsequentionalism holds that the consequences of an action are not the deciding factor but that something other than the consequences determines whether the action is right or wrong. Nonconsequentionalist theories often make use of the notion of duty. Most people believe, for example, we have a duty to keep our promises, to tell the truth, not to harm others, not to kill, and so forth. The circumstances surrounding or the consequences of an action do not affect the duty to do (or not to do) the action. Suppose we have a duty to tell the truth. This duty does not entail we should tell the truth when it is convenient to do so and lie when it is not. It entails we should tell the truth whether it is convenient or not.

One of the best known nonconsequentionalists was Immanuel Kant. Kant argued that if we do not tell the truth or keep our promises, people will learn that they cannot depend on what we say. He raised the question of what would happen if everybody made promises without intending to keep them. He pointed out that promising would lose its meaning. After all, what good are promises if people always break them? Accordingly, for a nonconsequentionalist like Kant, we should always keep our promises and always tell the truth. Our duties do not pivot on the results or ends.

In health care contexts, the notion of duty, a nonconsequentionalist notion, plays an important role. There is a point beyond which caregivers will not be pushed or will not bend. They take their duties seriously, and external considerations will not be allowed to undermine those duties. Yet nonconsequentionalism is not an absolutely rigid doctrine. Sometimes it is necessary to weigh and balance conflicting principles in order to resolve an issue. For example, it may be necessary to lie in order to avoid breaking a promise or hurting another person.

Ethical Pluralism and "Gourmet Ethics"

Consequentionalism and nonconsequentionalism may seem to be irreconcilable, and either approach by itself may seem inadequate given the complexity of many health care decisions. In fact, most people do not embrace one approach to the exclusion of the other; they adopt a sort of "ethical pluralism."

The goal of health care professionals is to achieve certain desired *results*. On the other hand, their *principles* are important to them. They act in certain ways because they believe it is their duty to do so—it is part and parcel of what it means to be a doctor or nurse or other health care professional. They feel obligated to be truthful and trustworthy and responsible to their patients no matter what the consequences. The overriding principle not to harm and to benefit the patient, for example, guides health care professionals in every set of circumstances. The circumstances at most affect how the principle is to be applied.

Health care professionals can be spoken of as "gourmet ethicists"; they take the best of consequentionalism and nonconsequentionalism to make decisions and set policies. They also use the tactic of comparing a given situation with similar situations in the past, which some refer to as "casuistry." Such comparison provides helpful guidance as well.

Framing the Issue

An important step in dealing with an ethical issue is "framing the issue." Framing the issue involves making an initial decision as to what the ethical issue, controversy, or dilemma actually is. It also involves deciding what the components of the issue are and how to set up the topics to be discussed. It can greatly facilitate later steps by ensuring the issue is given a clear, workable formulation.

The importance of framing an issue will be illustrated by examining the issue of abortion. Although not a burning issue

in postacute care, it does acutely illustrate how people can dig
in their heels and dogmatically hold their ground.

If one person takes the position that abortion is murder and
another takes the position that the choice to have an abortion
should not be fettered with restrictions, the likelihood of any
resolution (or even agreement on the way to present the issue)
is small. Facile formulations of a complex issue preclude better understanding as well as resolution of the issue. Framing
the abortion issue as a question of life versus choice will ob-
struct any move toward agreement. Framing it as a question
of life versus privacy (i.e., the right to privacy, which arguably
includes the right to determine what shall be done with one's
own body) may lead to success. In the latter case, whether life
begins prior to conception, at conception, at viability, or at
any other stage of pregnancy is irrelevant. The beginning of
life is a consideration that would come into play, not in the
framing of the issue, but in the process of addressing it and
trying to achieve a consensus.

Framing an issue, especially an emotionally charged issue,
provides a more dependable starting point for dealing with it.
When an issue is better formulated, the opposing sides, even
if they do not revise their views, will at least have a better understanding of what their own views are, as well as the views
they disagree with. In short, they will at the least be arguing
about the same issue. If an opponent is unwilling to play the
"framing game," it may be best to avoid further debate so as
to minimize frustration. Without this important step, people
tend to talk at cross-purposes or discuss different, perhaps
dramatically different, issues.

Recently, in one of my classes a student raised the "ethical
issue" of early discharge in delivery room settings. Although
there may be ethical issues associated with early discharge,
early discharge is not itself an ethical issue. Some of the concerns at stake have to be examined before we can frame this
issue in a way that will allow us to proceed along a clear path.
Cost containment, offering the best possible care, limited resources, and the like, initially come to mind. Perhaps the crux
of the issue should be viewed as a conflict between cost containment and offering the best possible care. However, this
formulation seems wrong because the "best possible" care
would supersede, if not preclude, considerations of cost.
Maybe "best possible" should be changed to "high-quality"

or even "appropriate" care. Also, is it cost containment that we are really talking about? Maybe we are really talking about "cost control" or "cost reduction." Framing the issue as "balancing the delivery of appropriate care against wishes to reduce costs" is more realistic and offers more hope that a consensus can be achieved.

Those given the responsibility of addressing ethical issues in a facility or agency or as members of an ethics committee should try to provide caregivers with the skills and knowledge they need to figure out what they should do. The goal is not to resolve controversies at all costs but to offer a forum for airing controversies, focusing on the issues at stake, and helping all involved arrive at sensible decisions.

Justifying Your Position

Once someone has made a provisional decision, the way in which he or she justifies the decision becomes an interesting process in itself. One of the most difficult things for the students of ethics to understand is what justifying a position means. The best way to determine whether a provisional decision is valid is to test its weakest components. The old adage that a chain is only as strong as its weakest link applies here.

In challenging a provisional decision, we examine whether its weaknesses are too great for us to live with the decision. If they are, we need to go back to work and find a superior one. We imaginatively construct circumstances or counterexamples that others might use to challenge our decision. By examining what might occur, we can arrive at a richer understanding of any complex problem and hopefully arrive at a good decision.

Justifying a decision is perhaps more important in ethics than many other fields because it is the main way of testing the decision and refining it. A clinical decision might be shown to be wrong if its medical consequences turn out to be harmful. An ethical decision does not allow this kind of test. It is shown to be a good or bad decision through the imaginative exploration of an array of consequences and alternatives.

The process of justifying an ethical decision also allows others to discuss, disagree with, challenge, or support the decision on the basis of knowledge. If the person justifying the decision claims to be motivated by a sense of obligation to do no harm, others involved in the decision will at least understand where the person is coming from. This creates an opportunity for refining, reformulating, and collaborating on the decision to achieve better results, which process itself might be helpful in evaluating the validity of the decision.

A similar process is operant in law. The result in a legal case will always pivot on a certain principle, rule, or interpretation. Perhaps a major difference between ethics and law is that law generally defines the outcome in advance. A lawyer will decide what outcome to pursue and will start from the outcome and work backwards, looking for the principle or rule that will support the desired outcome. In ethics, we start with the rules and principles and work toward an outcome—a defensible decision.

Rights and Wishes

The notion of right or rights deserves some attention, primarily because it is assigned such great importance by so many. Ethicists generally view rights as good things. Rights have great weight or authority and, like privileges, cannot be easily overridden or ignored. Rights are always presented as adversarial. Assertion of a right is always associated with a demand that others have a corresponding duty to act (or refrain from acting) a certain way and may be open to sanctions or penalties if they fail in their duty.

When clinicians talk about honoring rights, they really mean identifying the wishes, values, preferences, and directives of patients and acting in accordance with them. Talk of wishes and choices rather than talk of rights is perhaps more in keeping with the clinical setting. As a last resort, rights always can be invoked.

Of course, it is possible to argue that *rights* is the traditional term used in policy statements (e.g., The American Hospital Association Bill of Rights) and we should stick with this kind of language. One response is that tradition is not always a good guide, and that we should develop enforceable "rights."

When the Patient Self-Determination Act first came into effect, many facilities and agencies attempted to respond by informing people of their *rights* rather than assuring them their *wishes* would be acknowledged and supported. Yet complying with the spirit of the act is what is most important, not talking about rights and obligations. Setting a more positive tone by telling patients that their wishes will play an important role in shaping their care creates a more comfortable environment for them. Focusing on identifying and honoring wishes and values can transform what might otherwise be perceived as an unwanted and annoying compliance provision into a positive marketing and community relations tool.

Right and Wrong Answers

It is difficult if not impossible to "do ethics" if one lacks the appropriate information upon which to base decisions. The process of refining a provisional decision involves determining what information we need to make a better decision. As we test or weigh the decision, we look for its strengths and weaknesses and thereby uncover what needs clarification. By assessing a wide range of options and alternatives, we can arrive at a better decision, perhaps even the best.

Those who assert that there are no right or wrong answers miss the boat. Even those who assert that "it's all relative" must identify *what* is relative and why and then provide a justification for their position. An unexamined decision will always be inferior to one that undergoes refinement and upgrading. A refined decision is much more likely to resolve the issue being addressed. If an ethics committee is undertaking the refinement process, it is important for the members to remember that their primary goal, contrary to common opinion, is not to smooth over any conflict but to define the process of making a good decision (which hopefully, but not necessarily, will also settle any conflict).

ESTABLISHING A FRAMEWORK FOR DECISION MAKING

Establishing a framework for decision making is an important step in dealing with ethical issues. Many ethical concerns people have or wish to address or resolve can be interpreted differently from different perspectives. The fact that ethics committees are more often than not interdisciplinary testifies to the importance of diversity of perspective in handling problems composed of diverse components.

Many times when people claim that they have an ethical problem they want to address, what they really mean is that they want to determine what they can do with legal impunity. They disguise legal questions as ethical ones. Covering of one's backside has been and probably will continue to be a significant motivating factor in bringing issues to the attention of an ethics committee, since this type of committee is more accessible and less threatening than the hospital legal counsel or an outside attorney. (It also does not charge the petitioner by the hour!)

Therefore, an initial task is to identify why a given issue is being brought to the attention of the ethics committee and to sort out as best as possible the legal, ethical, clinical, and administrative components. This serves various purposes. (1) It minimizes use of the scattergun approach to problem solving (the wider the spread, the greater chance of being on target). When people are not sure of the nature of an issue and what tools are needed to address it, they may say it has legal, ethical, policy, and other implications just to be safe. This strategy will lead to the wasting of resources. (2) It allows a more accurate definition of the issue. (3) It breaks what might appear to be an overwhelmingly complex issue into simple components. (4) It allows committee members to better understand the issue, including relevant distinctions and misperceptions.

Whether the issue is primarily a legal or ethical issue, it still must be addressed. The patient and the doctor or other caregiver must make a decision together, or if the patient wishes are unknown or unclear and there is no advance directive and no appropriate surrogate, the doctor or other caregivers will have to act in the best interest of the patient. Some states have surrogacy laws dictating the order of decision makers to be used in the absence of a surrogate specifically designated in advance by the patient.

Creative problem-solving techniques can serve an institution well. Focused discussions offer opportunities for enriching caregivers' understanding and allow them to deal with problems that in the past they have been ill-equipped or reluctant to address. Such discussions can increase the comfort level of those involved and help them hold in abeyance their own moral preconceptions and prejudices and look at an issue in a clearer and more open minded way.

UNDERSTANDING PIVOTAL INGREDIENTS AND KEY CONCEPTS

It is important for caregivers to understand pivotal ingredients and key concepts that arise repeatedly in ethical contexts in health care in order to gain insight and comfort and develop better evaluative and decision-making tools. Becoming familiar with ethical, administrative, systemic, and legal concepts will increase their ability to address issues in a more proactive and comprehensive fashion.

Occasionally, ethical and legal issues so closely overlap they are almost indistinguishable from each other. In these cases, a process of uncovering the similarities of the issues while defining their distinctiveness can be important. Note that sometimes the same term is used differently or different terms are used identically by different professions. For example, an ethicist may speak of *autonomy* or *self-determination* and an attorney may speak of *privacy*. When the attorney is questioned, he or she may assert that the right to privacy encompasses the right to determine what should be done with one's own body (which sounds much like the self-determination of which the ethicist speaks). Similarly, the ethicist, when questioned about self-determination, may begin talking about the right to privacy. And of course the clinician may speak of values and the right to decide. All are dealing with the same issue.

INFORMED CONSENT AND KNOWLEDGE

Having a foundation of knowledge to build upon is essential for resolving the ethical issues we confront. To see this, consider the concept of informed consent. Informed consent is consent that has been given by someone who is demonstrably knowledgable about the risks entailed by the consent (e.g., the risks of a specific procedure the person has agreed to undergo).

Informed consent is sometimes treated as an ethical issue and sometimes as a legal issue, but in fact it is both. There are ethical and legal reasons for making certain that when someone agrees to a medical procedure or treatment, the person understands what is at stake and is not simply nodding his or her head to be amenable. Another way of looking at it is that the person must be informed of and have the capacity to understand the risks (and benefits) if consent is truly to occur. Knowledge and decision making necessarily go hand in hand.

KNOWLEDGE AND ETHICS

The idea that ethics and knowledge are closely, if not inextricably, linked is well rooted in the Western tradition. The ancient Greeks believed that knowledge and ethics were necessary to each other. How could one possibly make reliable decisions in the absence of pertinent information?

The Greeks distinguished different levels or stages of knowledge. The first and most primitive way of knowing is that of unexamined opinion, which the Greeks called *doxa*. This often involves the uncritical adoption of information and the uncritical acceptance of opinion as truth or knowledge. At this level, all opinions are considered to be of equal merit, everyone is entitled to his or her own opinion, and there is no court of appeal. Blind faith—strict adherence without examination—is standard procedure.

At the next level is what the Greeks referred to as *phronesis*. Phronesis is basically examined opinion. At the level of phronesis, people think through and improve their opinions. They try to achieve a richer understanding of what they have previously believed. Phronesis does not involve the same degree of certainty as scientific knowledge (i.e., knowledge that has been rigorously examined), but it is a step in the right direction.

Episteme is richer and more refined knowledge. Superior to doxa or phronesis, it is attained when we develop theories and carefully examine our preconceptions and past judgments using the best of our critical assessment and evaluative tools. It involves testing our provisional solutions and hypotheses and arriving at reasoned and well-founded judgments.

The highest form of knowledge for the Greeks was *sophia*, or wisdom. Sophia involves knowing how things fit together in the larger scheme of things. The Greeks believed few if any could achieve sophia in this life. (Unfortunately, sophia is the form of knowledge that would seem to be needed to understand and coordinate our health care system and establish its priorities.)

It is important to recognize that remaining on the level of opinion, especially unexamined opinion, is unsatisfactory. Addressing issues in a way that takes account of their complexity requires going well beyond prejudice, hearsay, innuendo, and misperception. By directing our focus at the more important root issues, we can evaluate what we are investigating or attempting to understand and then proceed to higher levels of knowledge. Although we may never exceed the level of phronesis in our determinations, at least we will not allow ourselves to be comfortably and uncritically entrenched at the level of doxa.

LEGAL AND ETHICAL CONCEPTS

Privacy and Self-Determination

The notion of privacy is rooted in common law. The right of privacy developed out of the concept of trespass, specifically trespass to chattels (property). Trespass, first defined in the context of property, like many common law concepts, was only extended to deal with persons as an afterthought, for matters of person were generally of less import to the courts than were matters of property. Trespass to persons was later redefined as *battery*. Battery means little more than unpermitted touching, an unpermitted violation of a person's privacy. Battery was construed as an insult to or a compromising of one's privacy. The invisible sphere that surrounds each person is legally protected from intrusions by others.

When people talk about privacy in health care contexts, they are really often talking about battery. Furthermore, they talk about privacy not so much as a protection but as a right— a right that encompasses the right of self-determination, the right to refuse treatment, and the right to die.

A right is something to which someone is entitled. It cannot be easily taken away, as can a privilege. A privilege generally has conditions attached to it, conditions that must be met if the privilege is to remain in force. The only way a right can be challenged or undermined is when it conflicts with another right, which may override it. The process of weighing conflicting rights against each other is directed toward arriving at a resolution to what might otherwise appear to be an irremediable problem. Each right is still viewed as valid, but one is seen as stronger than the other in this instance and thus the determinant of what is right to do.

The concept of autonomy, which occurs mainly in philosophical contexts, corresponds to the concept of self-determination used in legal contexts. In case law it was argued as early as 1914, in the Schloendorff case,[1] that "any individual of sound mind has the right to determine what shall be done to his own body." The concept of self-determination expanded over time to encompass the larger sphere of privacy, including not only bodily privacy but also psychological privacy. According to the concept of autonomy, a person should be free to do as he or she wishes.

One of the first steps in addressing ethical issues is to ensure consistency in the way similar topics are characterized and assessed. This includes assessing policies within a given facility to ensure consistency, continuity, and coherence. It is also important that the policies be congruent with the facility's mission. By evaluating the policies to see whether they meet these conditions, the facility's staff can reduce administrative frustration and devise clearer mechanisms to prevent and resolve conflicts. The staff should be familiar with pivotal ingredients in decision making and key concepts and criteria for addressing ethical issues before they take on this task.

As mentioned above, rights are adversarial in nature. They are essentially entitlements and are associated with sanctions or penalties levied against those who do not honor them. Not acting in accordance with rights can lead to serious consequences, including claims for financial damages.

People have a sense of private personhood that partially determines their values, wishes, and choices, and it is they who should decide what is done to them medically. If a patient is not capable of deciding this, a surrogate or substitute decision maker should act for the patient and tell caregivers what the patient said or would likely have decided were the patient able to decide. Significant problems may arise in such cases, especially when the patient's wishes are unclear or unknown. Determining decisional capacity becomes an important factor in honoring patient intent and identifying what is right or best for the patient.

Determining Decisional Capacity

It is important to highlight an inconsistency in determining decisional capacity. Many attorneys who have little experience working with health care facilities and little clinical exposure or sensitivity will assert that determining decisional capacity or competence is a legal matter and that persons are considered competent unless legally demonstrated in a court of law to be otherwise. In fact, the clinical determination of decisional capacity is an important part of the clinical enterprise and is a prerequisite for ensuring patient self-determination. I think it is appropriate to replace the word *competence* with *decisional capacity*, for while a patient may not be competent in the broad sense (e.g., may be unable to handle financial affairs) he or she may still possess the ability to appreciate the significance of a specific medical decision. In fact, the question at issue is whether the patient can understand and appreciate the significance of a specific medical decision *now*, not yesterday or tomorrow.

I have been repeatedly asked by psychologists and psychiatrists what can be done to prevent attending physicians from sending them patients to determine whether the patients are *competent* when the issue is whether they currently have the *capacity* to make a specific medical decision. If physicians asked that question instead of the question about competence, which is more complicated and difficult to answer, they would more often get the kind of answer they really need. (In fairness to physicians, psychologists and psychiatrists have a responsibility to contact the physicians for further clarification, a responsibility they do not always carry out.)

Fluctuating Capacity

Patients whose capacity is fluctuating can make binding decisions during periods when they are in a state of decisional capacity. Requiring a legal determination of capacity by a court for a patient with fluctuating capacity seems to be unduly burdensome and impractical. Imagine a scenario where a patient with fluctuating capacity must be reviewed by a court to determine his capacity. He would not necessarily be judged "incapacitated" but his thinking is not "always dependable and clear." Suppose he wakes up clearheaded and at that point has the capacity to make a medical decision but loses his capacity while being transported to the court. Later he regains his capacity but loses it again on the way back to the court. The patient might have to be transported back and forth repeatedly before the timing finally is right.

In a case of fluctuating capacity, having a court determine decisional capacity is unnecessarily cumbersome and a wasteful use of dollars at a time of limited resources.

Sometimes there are medical conditions that increase a patient's incapacity. The loss of potential for participating in ongoing decision making will be exacerbated if the patient becomes debilitated or sick as a result of going back and forth to a courthouse. This is a major reason why a clinical determination of capacity to make decisions is often acceptable in a wide range of circumstances. There are cases where a patient has a guardian but, in the estimation of a caregiver, has the capacity to make medical decisions. In such circumstances, clear and explicit documentation is critical.

The role of the caregiver also is critical. The caregiver must balance paternalism and autonomy. The caregiver is not vulnerable like the patient and possesses superior knowledge of the patient's condition and what it implies. Given this discrepancy in power, the caregiver has the opportunity to hinder or disable the patient. The flip-side of consent is always the integrity of the caregiver and the caregiver's willingness to honor patient wishes. What the caregiver should do is support and encourage self-determination on the part of the patient. When the patient consents to a procedure, the consent is an ingredient of the ongoing process of integrating the patient into the decision-making enterprise.

Advocacy

In this era of managed care, *advocacy* has become a buzzword. National health care trade organizations such as the American Medical Association are aware that the physician's traditional role as primary care provider is being challenged. They are encouraging patient advocacy and the physician's special qualifications to act as an advocate as a way of protecting both the patients' and physicians' interests.

In the past, the language of advocacy was used most often by members of the nursing profession, who were told that they must intercede on behalf of the patient when the physician was unclear or mistaken about the patient's wishes. The nurse's role was really that of facilitator, helper, interpreter, or guide.

The word *advocacy* is derived from the Latin term *advocare*, meaning to stand in someone's place and speak for that person. Lawyers are called advocates because they stand in for clients and argue on their behalf. Advocacy thus implied "replacing" the person for whom an advocate was speaking rather than supplementing or clarifying what the person had said. Some have argued that advocacy in the sense of standing in for another is a kind of paternalism. It seems to be based on an assumption that the patient is unable to speak for him- or herself and uses the supposed incapacity as a license to supplant the patient and remove the patient from the decision-making loop.

As used currently, however, *advocacy* means something quite different. Once the difference is understood, advocacy will be perceived as more important and more empowering than it was in the past. Whether one is a physician, physician's assistant, nurse, nurse practitioner, dietitian, social worker, or other health professional, patient advocacy is an essential component of the care process, especially because appropriate care is in jeopardy of being replaced with inferior and less costly care and access to services is becoming more difficult. The need for caregivers to be advocates has increased rather than decreased. Standing in a patient's shoes and arguing in favor of availability of services or negotiating with payors is an emerging challenge. The object is not to substitute one's judgments or choices for the patient's but rather to argue for or even demand appropriate treatment.

Unfortunately, clinicians may find that advocating for those they serve is not only increasingly important but even a necessary precondition of providing care. This is particularly the case when the best treatment for a patient is more costly than other standard treatments. The clinician needs to anticipate challenges by the insurer and act to protect the patient's interests.

Common Courtesy

In the past, many of the complex problems that arose in health services delivery and medical research were not addressed in an open forum, and medical ethics was a narrow field that focused on advertising, appropriate ways to dress, and the like. Professional etiquette was also an area of interest, but despite that fact there was little discussion of common courtesy.

Common courtesy is frequently ignored in busy environments or when a patient becomes absorbed into the care process as a result of undergoing a complex matrix of procedures.

For example, in an institutional setting, a group of curious onlookers, including staff, residents, and students, may enter the room of the "interesting patient" without any sensitivity to the fact that they are invading the privacy of the patient. The patient is poked and prodded and questioned for educational purposes. Rarely will a physician in a teaching facility take the time to extend the common courtesy of entering the patient's room before the rest of the group and asking in a noncoercive and nonintrusive way whether it is okay to bring in the others. A "no" answer should not generate recrimination or reprisal, and a "yes" answer should not be taken to obviate the need to balance educational benefit against patient privacy. Handling this matter well can transform a possibly annoying intrusion into a positive experience for the patient. Indeed, the patient might well end up feeling pleased at receiving the special attention.

The patient is already stripped of the dignity and control he may normally possess and is magically transformed from a person to a patient, that is, into a lesser being by virtue of mere admission into the institutionalized setting. Often he or she is assumed to be ill-informed and perhaps incapable of making responsible decisions. Of course, if the patient is incapable of making many decisions, the reason may simply be that the caregivers have not taken the time to provide the information needed for making responsible decisions. This does not give the caregivers license to avoid describing the patient's condition and treatment options to the patient and integrating the patient more comfortably into the setting. Surely, it does not permit the caregivers to make the patient feel more alien or helpless than he or she already feels or to deny the patient common courtesy.

In the home setting, discourteously asking the patient's family to get out of the way so that the health care professionals can have a private meeting often makes the family feel unneeded, unwanted, and helpless. This type of behavior is frankly rude. How a patient is treated—courteously or discourteously—is a subtle indication of how the caregivers perceive him or her. It can determine whether the caregivers are seen as helpers or as adversaries. Demonstrating common courtesy can enhance communication with patients as well as fellow practitioners, and its importance should not be overlooked as caregivers address the more complicated problems that arise in health care ethics.

Conflicts between Patients' Decisions and Caregivers' Preferred Treatments

Caregivers often become more paternalistic when their patients choose treatments or procedures other than what the caregivers believe is the best option or that the caregivers deem ineffective or harmful. In fact, questions as to whether a patient has the capacity to make decisions most often arise when the patient disagrees with what the physician or other caregivers want to do.

One way to diffuse bad feelings and avoid conflict in such situations is to be sensitive to and establish mechanisms for dealing with medical futility and anticipatory grief. Family members should be aware of both good and bad outcome scenarios and also be informed of how the patient is faring from day to day and from intervention to intervention. This sets the stage for discussion and communication and allows choices and anticipated decisions to be perceived as components of an ongoing process rather than discrete events. It also allows the family to be involved in a positive way rather than feel alienated and unneeded.

Caregivers should also be familiar with the relevant policies and procedures and document procedures clearly and comprehensively. As practice guidelines and standards and clinical pathways become more common, these can be integrated into the decision-making process and shared with the family and the patient, both in advance and when a specific circumstance arises. It is critical to involve the patient early on as a partner in the process of care and decision making. If there is a surrogate decision maker or the patient wants a family member or friend involved in decision making, this person should be treated as a full partner early on in the care process.

Futility

The issue of medical futility is increasingly being discussed in health care ethics and legal contexts. Futile procedures are those that provide no benefit to an individual other than prolonging the dying process. The issue arises when a person has suffered a serious insult for which there is no appropriate treatment and multisystem failure is occurring. Any last-ditch efforts will be futile and probably only will be performed because of an adamant request on the part of the patient or fear of potential legal liability for the failure to "do everything" on the part of the caregiver. The issue also arises when the natural course of a disease prohibits the caregivers from doing anything more than minimally pushing back the moment of death.

In cases of medical futility, the caregivers should focus on doing whatever is in the patient's best interests. Symptom control, keeping the patient out of pain, and ministering to the spiritual needs of the patient and the family are the most important goals. Creating mechanisms for dealing with anticipatory grief will be far more helpful than last-ditch tactics that do no good and could cause harm. Medical futility provisions will become more prevalent as the need to reduce the use of marginally beneficial services becomes greater.

Inadequate Care

Another important ethical issue in home care arises when a caregiver is providing inadequate or inappropriate care. What is the role of the home health care nurse in such a circumstance? Of the doctor? What policies and quality assurance mechanisms can be formulated to deal with this type of situation?

Caregivers sometimes become burnt out, suffer from excessive unresolved grief, have an alcohol or drug problem, or have some infectious disease that might pose danger to their patients. These types of situations also can be dealt with by policies that contain mechanisms for referral, support, and counseling as well as procedures to meet patients' needs while protecting their interests. Health care professionals must develop agency and facility policies to address these issues and discuss them more openly in educational institutions and national organizations responsible for developing health care standards.

TELEMEDICINE AND EMERGING COMMUNICATION TECHNOLOGIES

Telemedicine is playing an increasing role in the provision of health care services. It can be used for identifying problems, clearing up uncertainties, and educating patients and nonprofessional caregivers. It is an attractive supplement to hands-on care and can aid in filling the gaps in the continuum of care.

The ethical issues associated with telemedicine will increase in frequency and seriousness if telemedicine becomes used as a substitute for rather than a supplement to hands-on care and the intimacy of the caregiver-patient relationship.

Anything that distances the patient from the caregiver is negative; anything that enhances the relationship is positive. Telemedicine has the potential to do both. It provides a means of efficient and timely communication between the caregiver and the patient so that they can be active agents in a dynamic process of care. On the other hand, it can be used by the caregiver to avoid seeing the patient in order to reduce the cost of providing care. This tactic can compromise the quality of care.

The ability to use communication technologies for enhancing our ability to monitor our patients from a remote location can offer an important supplement for caring for them and for adding a sense of security for those who do not have the luxury of 24-hour in-home support. It can also be an extremely effective vehicle for forming support groups with other home care patients to develop a greater sense of community and create a network for those who suffer from common ailments. It cannot only provide an opportunity for sharing and benefiting from the experience others have in coping with their illness or circumstance but also minimize loneliness. It also offers an important sense of worth when one can share what one has experienced to minimize the uncertainty or fear of another. One can be helpful rather than helpless. For the caregiver telecare and telemedicine can be an invaluable aid for diagnosis assessment and intervention. For example, it can be a valuable resource for family members who may be uncertain about wound healing who can focus a videocamera on the wound site to show the clinician at a remote location who can communicate with them at the same time they are transmitting and can ask for additional information or zoom in for a closer look. Perhaps the most serious ethical issues in this domain deals with cost issues, specifically if telemedicine and telecare become a substitute rather than a supplement to hands-on care. Other cost concerns pivot on the willingness of a first- or third-party payer to provide or reimburse for needed audio-visual equipment in the home. Other ethical issues associated with telemedicine include questions of who manages the information with compliance on the part of the remote patient, licensure issues, and confidentiality issues.

Telemedicine has enormous potential for training and education, and it can easily be integrated into the caregiving process. Legal issues surrounding recordkeeping and confidentiality must be considered, but these generally will present little difficulty. Ownership, sale, fair market value, and fraud and abuse issues must also be addressed.

One potential problem is patient noncompliance. The caregiver has to trust that the patient is availing him- or herself of the information provided by phone, fax machine, or computer terminal. The patient may have faulty equipment that prevents total communication, may have a medical condition that interferes with his or her capacity to understand what is being transmitted, or may be simply unwilling to follow the doctor's orders. If the caregiver does not see the patient occasionally, the consequences of these obstacles to compliance may remain hidden.

CASE STUDIES

Case 1

Mrs. A. has been in a long-term care facility for 18 years following a severe stroke. Her family had thought the stroke was just another episode of drunkenness and thus had delayed taking her to the hospital for some time. Mrs. A. is able to feed herself and talk but does not possess the capacity to make medical decisions. In fact, her son has been her guardian for over 15 years.

For financial reasons, the long-term care facility arranges for Mrs. A. to move to another nongovernment nursing home.

Shortly after her transfer to the nursing home, she is rushed to the hospital with her trachea crammed with food. The emergency department clears the airway, but the medical resident evaluating her determines that she is probably in a persistent vegetative state. She is reddish colored and in flexion.

The medical resident informs her son that a persistent vegetative state is irreversible but fails to tell him that this is a complicated diagnosis that takes some time to establish with a reasonable degree of certainty. The son says that his mother would not have wanted her life prolonged and he states he wants no interventions. The medical resident asks if he could start an IV, and the son says no if the goal is only to extend the dying process. They agree together that no invasive procedures should be done. The patient's sodium level is close to 190 and her osmolality exceeds 400. The attending is mostly absent from the decision making, for she trusts the resident's judgment.

The resident informs the ethics consultant what he is doing since the consultant is involved in a study of persistent vegetative state patients. He tells the consultant that he is comfortable making such decisions and has had a good deal of experience with these kinds of cases. A dietitian becomes the source of greatest discomfort for the resident, for the dietitian feels that a decision to do nothing in such circumstances is wrong and contrary to her own practice and ethical guidelines. She urges someone to speak with the son and get his okay to initiate IV fluids to see if the patient's condition might change as a result of this minimally invasive intervention. After all, two weeks ago Mrs. A. had been sitting up and eating on her own.

The resident is encouraged by the ethics consultant to talk with the son. The resident tells the consultant to do it himself if he feels that strongly about it. The son is approached by the consultant, who says he understands the son's fears that his mother's life might be unnecessarily prolonged. But he also says it is important that the son know he is doing the right thing and has exhausted all reasonable alternatives. He assures the son that the resident, the attending, and the ethics consultant know what his wishes regarding his mother are. The son agrees to a few days of hydration to see if his mother's condition will improve. A 1000D bag is hung, and within several hours Mrs. A. is verbal. After she is stable, she is discharged to her son's house.

The home health nurse learns after some time that there is a great deal of guilt and unresolved grief on the part of all family members, who feel that had they taken their mother to the hospital more quickly she would never have been in this state.

- Should she approach the family to talk about this issue?
- Should she inform the physician and set some mechanism in place to address it?
- Since she has a closer relationship with the family, should she deal with it directly?
- What are the primary ethical issues in this case?
- If the son had denied use of IV fluids, should a court order have been sought?
- What duty, in terms of reversing hasty decisions, does the caregiver owe?

Case 2

A male HIV-positive patient is a prostitute who has been attempting to generate business during his stay in the hospital. He has solicited both staff and patients. His psychiatric evaluation indicates that he is sociopathic. He has repeatedly claimed he will continue to work as a prostitute, passing the virus to as many people as he can.

Suppose this man is discharged from the hospital to the home. The nurse caring for the patient has recently lost a family member to AIDS and is still grieving and angry. She is aware that the patient has rights, but she feels by helping the patient get better, she is helping him return to the streets and thus, cause harm to others. This serious dilemma, involving her individual conscience, is affecting her capacity to care for the patient.

- What is the ethical responsibility of the clinician who is primarily involved with this patient's care?
- What is the institution's responsibility to inform third parties (Department of Health), if any?
- Is there a broader social responsibility? If so, from where is it derived?
- What are the key ethical issues?

Notes

- What are the key legal issues?
- If the case was brought before an ethics committee, what should its recommendations be?
- Is it important to exhaust least restrictive alternatives before going outside of the facility?
- What role should individual conscience play?

REFERENCE

1. *Schloendorff v. Society of New York Hospital*, 211 N.Y. 125, 105 N.E. 92 (1914).

4

A Model for Making Better and More Justifiable Decisions

Many of the problems that arise in health care have multifaceted dimensions and require more sophisticated treatment than a facile application of personal values or beliefs. These problems are seldom neatly packaged; instead, they are complicated by legal, policy, or systemic considerations. Thus, in order to focus on the central issues, some process of sifting or isolating these issues is required.

The model described here, the Robbins Model for Decision Making and Isolating and Defining Ethical Issues,[1] is an organized format for assisting with complex decision making. Since problems have various degrees of complexity, the format is designed to be easily simplified or upgraded to adjust for individual circumstances. Although the model is not a cookbook of answers, it will serve as a framework for understanding issues and making decisions and will even suggest possible decision options. Figure 4-1 is a flowchart outlining the basic steps of the model. The following case example will demonstrate, step by step, how the model works.

A SAMPLE APPLICATION

The Given Situation

Mr. David is a 58-year-old patient with chronic obstructive pulmonary disease who undergoes surgery at a hospital. Because of complications, he suffers an anoxic event that renders him incapable of making medical decisions. He has informed his primary care physician and his wife on various occasions that if any problems resulted, he did not want to spend the rest of his life on a ventilator and he did not want life-prolonging medical procedures to be undertaken. He has initiated neither a medical durable power of attorney nor any other written or verbal advance directive.

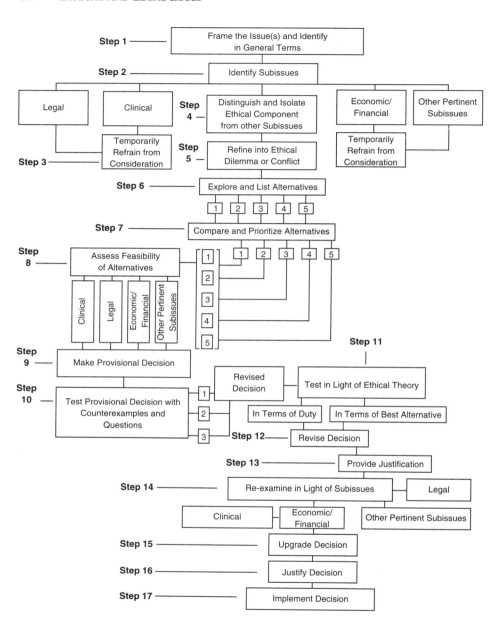

Figure 4-1 Flowchart of Decision-Making Model. *Source*: © Dennis A. Robbins. Adapted from The Robbins Model in T. Rando, ed., *Grief, Dying and Bereavement: Clinical Interventions for Caregivers*. Research Press, Champaign, Illinois.

The attending physician knows the family well but has recently become hyper-sensitive to the likely consequences of a malpractice suit and wishes to insulate himself from perceived potential liability. As a result, he is somewhat hesitant to act in accordance with what he thinks are the patient's wishes. He believes that by putting the patient on a ventilator he could save his life or at least reduce significant morbidity. What if the problem was something as simple as a mucous plug, which intubation alone would cure?

The wife is adamant that no measures be taken to extend her husband's life should he suffer cardiac or pulmonary arrest and assures her husband that she will be an advocate for him in the event that he will no longer be able to express himself. The patient's eldest son, an attorney, disagrees fervently and wants *anything* and everything to be done. There is intense family conflict as to what should or should not be done. Pastoral care and social services have attempted to resolve the conflict by means of a family conference, without success.

What should the physician do? What are his primary obligations? Should the family conflict or concerns about defensive medicine override the patient's wishes?

Determining What To Do

Step 1

Identify and frame the central ethical issues in general terms.

The central ethical issues to be faced in this situation can be stated in such questions as these: What are the rights of this now incapacitated patient? What obligations do the caregivers have to respond to and ensure the patient's rights and wishes? How can they identify the patient's wishes? How can they identify an appropriate surrogate decision maker. What is their responsibility to do so? Some discussion among the decision-making group on what rights or issues are at stake must occur before proceeding to the next step.

Step 2

Identify the subissues (these are often confused with the central ethical issues). This minimizes confounding factors and provides early identification of other pertinent issues.

There are legal, clinical, financial, and familial conflict subissues involved in this example. The legal issues include the patient's right to determine what shall be done to his own body (either by his own volition or, if he lacks capacity to express his wishes, through the decisions of a designated surrogate), the doctor's perception of potential liability, and the institution's liability. The clinical issue comes down to the question of what is feasible and appropriate from the medical perspective based on the prognosis, likelihood of reversibility of condition, practice guidelines or parameters, and so forth. Financially, the family is not well off, and the wife does not want to exhaust their meager savings. The familial conflict itself constitutes another pertinent subissue.

Step 3

Temporarily refrain from considering or weighing all subissues and focus on the central ethical issues.

Step 4

Distinguish and isolate the ethical component from other subissue components.

Legal and ethical issues often are confused and must be separated. Special care must be taken not to confound other pertinent subissues, such as administrative, cost, or systemic issues, with ethical issues. The ethical issues to be entertained in this case might include the following:

- the right to refuse treatment
- the right of self-determination (the right of the patient not to have his or her wishes compromised by external considerations)
- the physician's duty to his or her patient
- the conflicts surrounding intent and insulation from liability
- the responsibility of the facility administration
- the clarification of patient intent when financial considerations are involved and the ruling out of any "foul play" (e.g., a large life insurance settlement that might sway decision making on the part of the family)

- whether the physician discussed reversible conditions with the patient and the patient's views on such matters.

Step 5

Refine the ethical component by transforming it into an ethical dilemma. That is, state it as a conflict between at least two alternatives each of which has its strong points.

The central ethical conflict here involves a potential clash between the patient's rights and wishes and the right of the provider not to be placed in a compromising situation. The main question is whether the physician should honor "do not resuscitate" (DNR) orders or orders not to intubate (which is what the wife strongly favors) and risk a lawsuit brought by the son or try to manipulate the wife to agree with the son in order to avoid potential litigation.

Step 6

Explore and list alternatives for resolution of the ethical dilemma in an attempt to develop a provisional decision.

For purposes of illustration, four possible alternatives for the physician are suggested. (1) Motivated by duty, provide the best possible care in accordance with the patient's wishes while remaining within the boundaries of the law. (2) Intellectually feint and lie to the son and wife when medical procedures are performed. (3) Ignore both the wife and son and do what seems best medically. (4) Do whatever is possible to maximize protection from legal liability for oneself and the hospital.

Step 7

Compare, prioritize, or grade alternatives. This step can be adjusted as the complexity of problems increases. In grading alternatives, consideration may be given to conflicts between subissue components to further clarify each component. Also, at this stage some alternatives can be discarded and others can be revised or added. Assume that in this particular case there is a consensus that deceiving the wife or the son would be unreasonable and unacceptable. Also assume that there is a consensus that the physician should act in the best interests of his patient and write the DNR orders. That would, therefore, be the preferred option. The second option would be for the physician to insulate himself from liability and examine what documentation and other internal actions might be undertaken to prevent future problems while still honoring the wishes of his patient. Therefore the alternatives would be graded as follows: (1) honor the patient's wishes, (2) insulate against legal liability, (3) ignore the wife and son and do what is best medically, and (4) deceive the wife and son.

Of these four, the only real alternative anyone is comfortable with is the first, yet those who are making the decision may feel that a still better alternative might be available. And at this point they could choose to include that alternative (e.g., the alternative might be to consult the hospital's ethics committee and request it to assist in adjudicating the conflict that exists). For purposes of simplification, however, assume that the decision-making individuals adopt the first option.

Step 8

Assess the feasibility of the alternatives. This allows considerations of time, staffing, economics, legal constraints, and related issues to be integrated into the decision-making process.

Since in this case option 1 is by far the most obvious choice, it will not be necessary to assess the feasibility of each alternative. However, in other circumstances it may be appropriate to assess each alternative. Assessing feasibility includes focusing on clinical, legal, financial, and other pertinent components. For instance, is it medically feasible or appropriate to do this? Is this action consistent with legal standards or hospital policy or bylaws? There are financial and economic considerations in this particular example, and they should be assessed to determine if they have any bearing on the decision-making process at this stage.

Step 9

Make a provisional decision on the basis of the assessment of earlier steps. This is a summarizing step.

An upgraded decision that incorporates the clinical, legal, financial, and policy perspectives can be made. The provisional decision will likely be that the physician should act in the best interests of his patient and write the DNR order, but because of legal concerns and the desire of the wife not to exhaust all resources, turning the patient over to another caregiver or arranging another family conference are options that may help minimize his fear of potential liability. These options could be charted accordingly. The upgraded provisional decision would allow for providing the most appropriate care for the patient but at the same time would include mechanisms for insulating against potential liability.

Step 10

Test the provisional decision by constructing counterexamples. The purpose is to refine or upgrade the provisional decision. If the provisional decision does not withstand the challenges the counterexamples pose, it may be necessary to go back to earlier steps.

The following counterexamples and questions might apply to the case at hand: (1) Is it right for a physician to utilize other caregivers and the facility's resources and cause the family to exhaust its financial resources for the sole purpose of protecting against potential liability? (2) Does the introduction of nonmedical issues compromise medical care? (3) Should the decision be taken to court so that the physician can be absolved of all decision-making responsibility? (4) Isn't the principle that we should "save life at all costs" inconsistent with the writing of DNR orders? (5) Or what about the claim that without a consensus or guidance of a designated agent or surrogate we should "err on the side of life"?

Step 11

Test the upgraded decision in light of different ethical theories. Consider, for example, the decision from the perspective of a nonconsequentionalist theory, where the focus is on duty, and a consequentialist theory, where the focus is on the results of the decision. The purpose is to understand what two or more ethical theories might offer as potential solutions. In this step, it is also possible to apply a given ethical posture that a particular institution has already adopted as part of its policy.

Assume that only two ethical theories will be used to test the provisional decision: a nonconsequentionalist theory and a consequentionalist theory. Because of the nonconsequentionalist focus on duty or professional responsibility, the question might arise as to why patients come to physicians in the first place. The obvious answer is that they come to receive care and they assume that the physicians will do whatever is in the best interests of the patients and will not compromise the care provided because of external considerations (e.g., protection against legal liability). Physicians and other caregivers thus arguably have a duty to act in accordance with the wishes and intent of the patient.

In the case at hand, since the physician knows the family, and since the wife has been clear about her husband's intent, the physician's major responsibility lies with the patient, and if, in his judgment, the wife is providing a consistent and accurate account of what the patient had said were his wishes, that should be sufficient. The physician does not require (nor does the law) that there be a consensus among all the family members or surrogate decision makers although the law might outline a specific priority of decision makers. Controversial situations where the patient's wishes are unknown or unclear may require consensus among certain members of a class (e.g., brothers or sisters) when said class is the highest priority. The physician's responsibility is to act in accordance with professional standards and the wishes of the patient so long as the patient's wishes are not dramatically inconsistent with the ethics of the profession. The patient's survivors may sue, but to act in opposition to the patient's wishes or intents is a violation of duty. Of course, the physician also has a duty to be aware of the hospital's potential malpractice liability and to take steps to minimize it. This may involve contacting the hospital risk manager or an attorney to find out how to document the patient chart to insulate against potential liability as well as using proven conflict resolution techniques. However, the previously mentioned duty of providing the best care to the patient overrides this duty. To examine the decision from a consequentionalist perspective, those making the decision would try to imaginatively construct viable options and consider the consequences of each (including the provisional decision). The option having the best likely consequences would probably be picked as the best alternative.

The results of the assessment of both ethical theories would then be considered and the decision revised accordingly. In our example, we will assume that it will not be necessary to revise the decision significantly.

Step 12

Make a revised decision as a result of the previous step.

Step 13

Provide justification for the decision. Explain why it was chosen over the other options and why it is an acceptable decision.

The revised decision in the example might be justified by pointing to the fact that it has been tested against counterexamples and looked at from the perspective of different ethical theories and has held up, needing only minimal modification (which has further strengthened it).

Step 14

Re-examine the decision in the light of subissues. Consider each subissue component separately, then all components jointly. The purpose is to address the subtleties of the particular case.

In our example, modifications are not necessary.

Step 15

Upgrade the decision. In other words, revise the provisional decision to incorporate the results of considering the subissues.

If there had been modifications in Step 14, the decision would have been revised. Since there were none, this step can be omitted.

Step 16

Provide justification for the decision, this time including the subissues, some of which may be so significant that they modify the earlier decision radically. Construct counterexamples and test with theory.

In our example, the justification provided in Step 13 will suffice, since Steps 14 and 15 did not lead to a revision of the decision. If they had, a justification of the revised decision would have been attempted using counterexamples and different ethical theories.

Step 17

Apply and implement the decision in the clinical context.

This model can be a helpful aid and assist the user in becoming more adept at addressing a wide range of ethical issues. It can be used as a tool as well as an educational resource for developing problem-solving skills and techniques.

CASE STUDIES

Case 1

Mr. and Mrs. B. are a bright, financially successful middle-aged couple. Mrs. B. is terminally ill with a severe metastatic disease. She is in the hospital but she makes a point of keeping well groomed. She wears a beautiful robe and always has on her makeup. One day a nurse walks into the room and sees that she has not put on her makeup, her mouth is wide open, and she is staring aimlessly at the ceiling. It looks like the end is near. It is extremely hard on Mr. B. to see his wife in such a situation. One of the nurses who has been intimately involved in the case takes the husband aside and encourages him to go home and get some sleep. She assures him that he will be called if anything changes in his wife's condition. The nurse, after she leaves at the end of her shift, is away from the hospital for three days attending an out-of-town conference.

When the nurse returns, a colleague smilingly tells her to go see Mrs. B. "How is she?" asks the nurse. The reply is, "See for yourself." "Why the grin?" the nurse asks. "Well, the patient thinks you are having an affair with her husband," her colleague replies. The nurse is devastated, for she thought Mrs. B. trusted her. How could she have gotten this bizarre and totally wrong idea?

The nurse walks to the room and finds Mrs. B., last seen depressed and seemingly in the throes of death, now animated and smiling. When asked where she has been, the nurse responds by saying, "I've been out of town at a conference." "Indeed," Mrs. B. replies with a grin.

The nurse feels terrible but in her judgment the patient is happy and she decides not to raise the topic of the rumor. She leaves the room without saying anything about it, and later develops a plan to deal with the situation. Before she can act, however, she learns Mrs. B. has suddenly died. At an opportune moment she approaches the husband and tells him she is extremely sorry for the misunderstanding. Mr. B. says, "Don't be. My wife was happy believing that I was being taken care of in that way. Our sexual relationship was a very important component of our marriage. Thank goodness you didn't tell her it wasn't true."

- Is truth telling a good in itself?
- Is it okay to avoid the truth when it causes discomfort or pain?
- What role do the consequences of an act play in determining whether it is right?
- What role does professional responsibility play in this scenario?
- What are the major ethical issues in this case?

Case 2

Mr. J. has a metastatic cancer and has been hospitalized for eight weeks. Mr. J. wants desperately to go home and be with his family for his remaining days. His wife joins him in pleading with the doctor to do everything he can to release her loving husband from the hospital, but the doctor is not having a great deal of success getting Mr. J.'s pain under control.

A new morphine pump is able to finally provide more or less constant pain relief. When Mrs. J. learns her husband will get his wish and be able to return home, she smiles lovingly at her husband. What is totally unexpected is her reaction after she leaves the room with the doctor. When she is out of sight of her husband, she tells the doctor firmly that if her husband is sent home, she'll go crazy. There is no way she wants him home.

- Should the doctor inform the patient of this event?
- What are the central ethical issues that the doctor must confront as a result of the wife's response to the news?
- What responsibility, if any, does the doctor have to the patient's wife?
- What responsibility does he have to the hospital?

Case 3

Mr. R. is an 86-year-old man who has never been quite the same after the loss of his wife several years ago. His daughters are in denial about his condition and about what he really wants. He is reluctant to talk about his wishes to the doctor or nurse and is unwilling to even discuss the possibility of filling out an advance directive. Neither does he want to talk about the realities of his condition. He says he just wants a "tune up."

Mr. R. has a long history of diabetes, congestive heart failure, and heart disease and is now experiencing kidney problems. His physician has made recommendations to one of the daughters regarding what should be done given his deteriorating condition and the likelihood of multisystem failures. The daughter explains to him the realities of his condition, and although he becomes upset, he recognizes that decisions have to be made.

The physician is given the authority to write a DNR order for Mr. R. The home health nurse caring for him has very strong convictions about DNR orders, however, and she attempts to convince the patient to change his mind. This confuses him and he becomes depressed and angry with his physician. In fact, he says he wants another physician.

- If the nurse disagrees with the decision to write a DNR order and feels it is inappropriate for whatever reason, how should she try to effect a change?
- Who is responsible for an ethical decision of this sort?
- Would an ethics committee be helpful in resolving the case at hand?
- What are the main ethical issues in this case?
- How might conflict resolution policies help in this instance?

REFERENCE

1. Robbins D. A Decision-Making Model. In: Rando T, ed. *Grief, Dying and Bereavement: Clinical Interventions for Caregivers.* Champaign, Ill: Research Press; 1984.

5

Tracing the Legal Legacy surrounding Consent and End-of-Life Decision Making: From Quinlan to Cruzan

THE RIGHT OF PRIVACY

The United States Supreme Court has clearly stated that every competent adult has the right to control what happens to his or her body. This right is almost completely unfettered and only gives way when the state has an overriding interest in seeing medical treatment carried out, such as a blood transfusion for a parent with minor children. Barring those rare instances where the state's right outweighs the individual's interest, any treatment offered to a competent adult individual may be legally refused. This is true despite the wishes of family, friends, doctors, and even guardians.

There is a long-standing tradition in medicine that physicians must do everything medically possible to keep the patient alive. In recent years, the issue of allowing or even helping the patient to die has been opened up to vigorous debate. At present, do not resuscitate orders are commonplace. Courts have upheld the right of patients to refuse life-sustaining treatment in over 130 cases, and the U.S. Supreme Court has indicated that a right to refuse life-sustaining treatment can be found in the U.S. Constitution.

> The advance of life saving technologies has also contributed to the increased attention to medical decisions that lead to the death of patients . . . . Medicine now has the capacity to intervene and forestall death for almost any case. The Office of Technology Assessment Task Force estimated that in 1988 . . . 6,575 persons were dependent on mechanical ventilation and 1,404,500 persons were receiving artificial nutritional support.[1]

There has also been an attempt to legislate morality in this domain through legal decisions, most of which have attempted to shift decision

making back to the clinical forum, where it should have occurred in the first place. Twenty years have passed since the
Quinlan case was argued and a decision was reached, and
confusion still exists about what the decision means. Therefore, a short excursion into patient intent and the issues of
privacy and consent is in order.

Competent patients, as an extension of their right of privacy, must give permission for any medical intervention.
Expressed in another way, the patient must consent to allow
persons to perform procedures which, in the absence of consent, would not otherwise be permitted. In fact, from a legal
perspective, consent confers a legal privilege on health care
professionals to perform in a way that, in the absence of consent, would constitute a battery, which is simply the unpermitted touching of one person by another.

Thus, competent persons have the constitutional right to
consent to or to reject treatment. Incompetent persons in a
sense also have this right, although consent to or rejection of
treatment in their case is determined through surrogacy or
advance directives. Involvement of a surrogate decision
maker creates more complications than when the patient is
competent or has signed an advance directive, but the rights
of all patients must be respected.

The question arises, what is competency? The definition of
competency varies from state to state, but there is an emerging consensus. So long as an individual has the capacity to
understand the consequences of accepting or refusing medical treatment, that individual is competent for the purpose of
making medical decisions. This level of competency is now
generally referred to as *decisional capacity,* and it is usually determined by the attending physician. In some states, agreement by a second physician who has personally examined the
individual is also required. This concept of decisional capacity
has had an impact on many legal paradigms, especially when
applied to guardianship.

When patients are unable to speak for themselves, others
may exercise judgment in their stead and on their behalf. Substitute decision makers try to make the same choices that the
patients would have made had they been competent. If there
is no substitute decision maker and the physician knows the
patient's wishes, he or she can act on the basis of that knowl-

edge. In the absence of such knowledge, guardianship issues arise.

GUARDIANSHIP

The basic legal remedy employed when an individual can no longer take care of him- or herself is guardianship. Previously, a guardian of either person or estate was appointed for an individual who was determined by a court proceeding to be "incompetent." Competency was defined as the ability to make or communicate decisions about one's person or estate. The guardianship procedure is set up under the various state probate codes dealing with the passing of property at death and continues to be biased toward the issue of determining heirship.

A guardian can be appointed, however, after only a cursory review of the individual's true mental status. A physician is nominally appointed to determine competency and issues a one- or two-sentence summary report to a judge who never sees the individual whose competency is questioned. The individual's capacity to make personal decisions on a daily basis is not examined. The issue is simply too sensitive for most judges to deal with and so they ignore it. In fact, many people may not be capable of handling their financial affairs but may still be able to indicate whether or not they want a limb amputated. They have decisional capacity even though a court has determined that they need the protection of a guardian over their person or property.

Additionally, the definition of competency does not clearly address the issue of minors. Traditionally, minors, usually defined as individuals under 18 or 21 years of age, have not been legally capable of making decisions for themselves. "Emancipated minors" are exceptions to the rule—individuals who are at least 16 and are living independently. However, clearly children as young as 10 or 12 can understand the consequences of many medical decisions, and it can be anticipated that courts will therefore extend decisional capacity to minors.

Being placed under someone's guardianship is perhaps the most restrictive thing that can happen to a person. It implies that the person has no capacity or authority to make any decisions. Of course, there are times when a guardian is needed to act in the best interests of someone who is incapacitated or in some context cannot make an informed and reliable decision. Therefore, many jurisdictions are engaged in creating less oppressive and less restrictive forms of guardianship that are oriented toward a specific area of competence and are limited in some specific way. A guardianship, for example, may be limited to a certain range of decisions (e.g., medical or financial decisions) and it may also be limited in time (e.g., only in force during a period of recuperation from an illness).

The guardians are required to try to choose the decisions their wards would have made or, if they lack the necessary information, to choose decisions that are in the wards' best interests. A serious problem can arise when guardians are involved in the end-of-life decision making. It is not unusual for banks or other financial institutions to act as guardians. Such institutions often become extremely uncomfortable when faced with end-of-life decision making. They will often look to the family, which is fine. What isn't fine is when they fail to fulfill their duty as guardians and prolong the process of dying because of their failure to take those steps for which they are responsible.

PATIENTS LACKING DECISIONAL CAPACITY

When a patient has told the caregivers what he or she wants, their responsibility is to act in accordance with both the standards of the health care profession and the wishes of the patient. If the patient becomes incompetent, his or her wishes may be undermined by the family's own desires. For example, the family may take the position that mom has always been unrealistic in this domain (meaning they do not agree with her about this particular matter). The caregivers then are torn between honoring the wishes of the patient and carrying out the family's wishes (because it is the survivors who might sue). Their dilemma is not one of weighing battery against negligence (for failure to act) but of weighing the right of self-determination against the risk of litigation.

Ambiguity about who has the authority to make decisions for incompetent patients whose wishes are unknown continues to cause discomfort among clinicians. Dealing with patients who lack decisional capacity and have not indicated their wishes is particularly complex when the issue is whether treatment ought to be undertaken or withheld. The legal standards in this domain often have to be unbundled before they can be applied to a particular case. They are derived from several key legal decisions as well as from standards promulgated by the President's Commission on Ethical Issues in Biomedicine and Biomedical and Behavioral Research and the American Medical Association's Council on Ethical and Judicial Affairs.

THE COMMON LAW BACKGROUND

Treating the right to refuse treatment as an extension of the right of privacy is not new. As early as 1914, *Schloendorff*[2] said that "every human being of adult years and sound mind has a right to determine what shall be done with his own body."

Since 1976, such major cases as *Quinlan, Saikewicz, Dinnerstein, Spring,* and *Eichner v. Dillon* have provided guidelines for making decisions on behalf of incompetent patients. They have assisted caregivers in deciding the significance of a prognosis of hopelessness (*Quinlan*), determining what incompetent persons would likely have decided for themselves (*Saikewicz*), charting do not resuscitate (DNR) orders in advance (*Dinnerstein*), and identifying whether there is a need to approach the courts for prior approval (*Eichner v. Dillon*). These and other cases are discussed in detail below.

LEGAL CASES INVOLVING THE WITHHOLDING/ WITHDRAWING OF LIFE-PROLONGING MEDICAL PROCEDURES

In re Quinlan

The first important case in this area was *Quinlan*.[3] Karen Ann Quinlan, a 21-year-old woman, stopped breathing for two 15-minute periods for reasons not clearly identified. She was taken to an emergency department, where she was resuscitated and put on a ventilator. The hope was that temporary ventilatory support would start her on a return to normality. However, it was initially determined that she was comatose and later determined that she was in a persistent vegetative state.

This state is characterized by eyes opened unconsciousness, and destruction of most of the cerebral cortex. Initial trauma to the brain may cause the vegetative functions of the lower brain not to operate properly, in which case technological supports, such as a ventilator, are needed. Generally after three or four days, once swelling is reduced and the brain stem regains homeostasis, vegetative functions resume. The goal of the emergency department and of the hospital departments that treated Ms. Quinlan subsequently was to return her to normality and reduce significant morbidity by prompt and efficient interventions.

Although Karen Quinlan was put on a ventilator to increase her vital capacity and strength in hopes of reversing her plight, when it appeared that the goal of reversibility was not likely, questions arose as to what should then be done. For example, should she be kept on the ventilator if it was only going to prolong the dying process?

Some have argued that most ethical issues in medicine are consequences of technology run rampant. They seem to want to place the blame on technology and thus try to exonerate those who use it. Although it is true that technology presents many challenges, it also creates exciting opportunities. It is our failure to address the ethical issues that is the problem, not the technology.

Interestingly enough, our way of dealing with ethical issues in the United States reflect the Anglo-Saxon tradition of using the law to solve problems. When something is wrong, we say, "There ought to be a law" rather than "What can we do within the limits of ethical propriety?"

In *Quinlan*, the court attempted to solve the problem creatively. The court asked the doctors about the medical and ethical propriety of withdrawing mechanical ventilation. There was a question of whether the withdrawal of the ventilator would contravene the ethical standards and integrity of the medical profession.

The case was eventually decided by the New Jersey Supreme Court. The chief justice had the reputation of being an excellent problem solver. He had learned of an article about decision making and infant care review committees that suggested a committee forum was effective for addressing complex issues. He indicated that issues like the one in question could best be solved in the clinical arena but that having some mechanism in place to assist in the decision-making process, such as an ethics committee, would be appropriate. An ethics committee had the advantage that it would disperse responsibility among the committee members (not a goal we often seek in clinical consultations). The chief justice warned against using the courts for decision making, which the chief justice felt would "constitute a gratuitous encroachment upon the medical profession."

The so-called ethics committee in *Quinlan* was essentially a medical prognosis committee composed entirely of physicians. Their goal was to determine the medical prognosis, a fundamental ingredient in the decision-making process. The court indicated that the duty to treat diminishes as the prognosis dims and that in a hopeless case there is no need to continue extraordinary treatment. Thus, the ventilator could be removed if there was no likely chance of improvement. It was believed that as soon as the ventilator was removed she would surely die. Instead, Karen Ann Quinlan survived and remained in a persistent vegetative state for almost 10 years. (It was later discovered that the longest period someone had remained in a persistent vegetative state was 37 years, 111 days.)

At the time of *Quinlan*, little was known about persistent vegetative state. Quinlan's attorney, with whom I have shared a podium on many occasions, once indicated to me that had he known what he knows now about the condition, Quinlan would not have had to be in a nursing home in flexion for 10 years. A lot of agony and suffering could have been averted. Of course, we all have to do the best we can with the knowledge available at the time. It is pointless to flagellate ourselves for what is not yet known about the nature and natural history of all diseases or undiscovered techniques. Still we feel we should do more. It is a peril of the health care profession. Hopefully, the legacy of this young woman will save others from the same plight.

In 1990, almost 15 years after the Quinlan decision, I lectured in the Soviet Far East on end-of-life decision making to approximately 400 Soviet health care professionals. The isolated region, ten time zones from Moscow, was the locus of many of the Stalin-created gulag prisons. Interestingly, during the lecture I learned that everyone knew about Karen Ann Quinlan. They didn't know about third-generation antibiotics or good infection control and antiherpal medications, but they knew the intricacies of the Quinlan case. The case obviously had reverberations across the globe.

What one of the Russians said to me gave me a flash of insight. He politely told me that the fundamental difference between the way we practice medicine and nursing in the United States and the way the Russians practice is quite dramatic. Sometimes they have no technology, so they can only use their heads. They felt that in the United States medical personnel of various sorts are more comfortable using technology than their heads. Technology cannot dictate appropriate medicine, for medicine is an art of caring. Technological tools can help but not replace our judgment.

Superintendent of Belchertown State School v. Saikewicz

The next case that had dramatic national impact was a case that arose in Massachusetts involving a 76-year-old man who was a public ward in a state mental health facility.[4] Saikewicz had a mental age of 2 years and 10 months and an IQ of less than 50. He had been institutionalized for 53 of his 76 years. He had two sisters but he had little relationship with them. He suffered from myeloblastic leukemia, and the only intervention that was thought to have a chance of helping him was chemotherapy. The question was whether to administer it to him. Since patients have to give their consent for such a procedure a problem arose, for he did not possess the decisional capacity to give such a consent. He had been in a circumstance of enforced helplessness due to his institutionalization and also lacked the capacity to understand and appreciate the significance of the information he would need to make a responsible informed and voluntary decision.

The Massachusetts Supreme Court suggested that the focus should be on the patient's wishes. The standard to be used was that of substituted judgment. Basically, this standard entails that decisions made for someone be consistent with "what this individual would likely have decided were he able to decide for himself." Since we all have different perceptions and points of view, the court-appointed guardian was to determine what would be consistent with Saikewicz's views and what would be in his best interests. The guardian ad litem, that is, the guardian appointed for the purpose of the litigation, had to consider what someone Saikewicz's age would likely do. He believed that most people in similar circumstances would likely elect to undergo the therapy. However, the guardian also had to consider what Saikewicz in particular would likely have decided if he had possessed decisional capacity. Given his inability to understand what was being done to him and why, instead of hope, Saikewicz would probably experience only fear and pain. He might even perceive the treatment as a punishment. Consequently, the guardian thought it would be inappropriate to administer the chemotherapy. The substituted judgment standard requires the surrogate decision maker to choose, not what most people would likely want or what the surrogate would want, but the alternative that *this specific individual* would likely have chosen.

This was a very sensitive decision. One year after *Saikewicsz* had been decided, Chief Justice Liacos of the Massachusetts Supreme Court wrote up the case. In the process he took some creative liberties. He in fact took aim at the New Jersey court that had decided *Quinlan*. That court had said that the courts should not routinely become involved in such matters, for their involvement would "constitute a gratuitous encroachment upon the medical profession." The response of Chief Justice Liacos was that "rather than constituting a gratuitous encroachment, these cases require the dispassionate investigation of the court consistent with the spirit upon which this judicial branch of government was created." His opinion was criticized by many as an overstepping of proper bounds. He seemingly went beyond the main issue and indicated that going to court was the best way to ensure that the wishes of incompetent patients were met. The reaction to his decision was enormous, and he was flooded with letters loaded with frustration from clinicians and others.

In re Dinnerstein

Within two months another case, *In re Dinnerstein*,[5] arose in Massachusetts that clarified *Saikewicz*. Shirley Dinnerstein suffered from late-stage Alzheimer's disease. One of her sons, a physician, was serving as her substitute decision maker. The patient asked that a DNR order be written in advance as an extension of the substituted judgment standard. This case was heard by a judge who was a hospital trustee.

Dinnerstein was the first case in America to deal with the issue of writing a DNR order in advance. The decision supported this strategy as an extension of the substituted judgment standard outlined in *Quinlan* and *Saikewicz*. Unfortunately, many were confused as to what to do after Chief Justice Liacos, in *Saikewicz*, had indicated that it might be necessary to go to court to have decisions like this made. Instead of sensible DNR orders, a large array of codes were devised: Dr. No heart codes, code 250s, code 500s, designer codes (sky blue, light blue, etc.), gentleman codes, slow codes, and the like. Caregivers were also unclear about what DNR meant. DNR, which refers only to withholding cardiac and/or pulmonary resuscitation, was mistaken to encompass all kinds of other supports and treatment modalities.

In re Spring

Not willing to leave well enough alone, the Massachusetts Supreme Court took another shot at resolving autonomy issues in its decision in *In re Spring*.[6] Earle Spring, like Quinlan and Saikewicz, was incompetent. Spring stubbed his toe, which became infected and later necrotic. When he finally sought medical attention, he was put on a regimen of antibiotics and experienced renal failure. He then went on dialysis and perhaps developed dialysis dementia or aluminum toxicity (it was never clear which was the case). I had the chance to speak with the attending on this case and also worked with one of the court-appointed physicians, who said that the reason this case got to court was that the hospital learned the son was considering suing his employer. Since the son "had lawyer contacts," the hospital decided it ought to "have this looked at more carefully." Perhaps because of Spring's medical problems, his wife had a stroke, and she was in a long-term care rehab facility while he was in the hospital. Meanwhile, his son was attempting to be appointed guardian so he could end the dialysis. The court wanted to retain control, and a cumbersome legal process ensued.

The court set forth 13 different factors to be used in decision making. Interestingly enough, except for the patient's wishes, these were all medical criteria. The factors included what clinicians should consider in their assessment, such as risks, benefits, diagnosis, and prognosis. However, exactly how these were to be integrated into decision algorithms and matrices was unclear, as was the question of what weights should be assigned to the 13 variables. Would the patient's

wishes count a lot or a little? Five percent? Twenty-five percent? What about the prognosis? Rather than clarifying the issues, the Spring criteria caused discomfort, confusion, and
absurd delays. The *Spring* decision itself came almost two
years after Spring's death. An emergency in a hospital or
nursing home calls for immediate action. The courts move at a
snail's pace. Incredible as it sounds, judges in Massachusetts
at that time were considering carrying beepers to be more
readily available. This is not meant to suggest that the courts
cannot be helpful and timely in dealing with emergency
guardianship. However, there is no need for them to meddle
in cases like Spring's where family members are available
which should have been handled in the clinical forum. Also,
clinicians need to be more sensible in how they deal with decision-making responsibilities. The fact that the son knew some
lawyers should not have made any difference, other than perhaps more careful documentation to assuage the physician's
discomfort.

In re Eichner and *Eichner v. Dillon*

The next important case was *In re Eichner*.[7] Brother Fox, an
86-year-old religious cleric (who used to teach medical ethics),
was lifting a flower box on his roof when he suffered an in-
guinal hernia. He went to the hospital for routine hernia repair, but because of problems encountered during the surgery
he suffered an ischemic event that rendered him
encephalopathic. Fox had both a biological and religious family, and together they agreed that Father Eichner, his religious
superior, would act for him. Eichner, as surrogate decision
maker, attempted to have Fox's ventilator removed. However, Dennis Dillon, the district attorney of Suffolk County,
New York, felt that the state had an obligation to protect life at
all costs and mandated a five-point certification process that
had to be undertaken to ensure the wishes of the incompetent
were respected. The process involved a mock adversarial legal proceeding, a court-appointed physician, and an ethics
committee of three physicians, among other things. Eichner
sought a more reasonable alternative and approached the
New York State Court of Appeals,[8] which said that "any reasonable indication of patient intent will suffice and that there
was no need to approach the court to determine the propriety
of these kinds of decisions." When someone is dealing with

the loss of a loved one or a friend, we don't need to disenfranchise the patient nor to bludgeon his or her substitute decision makers with a mock adversarial process, particularly when the patient's wishes are so clear.

WITHHOLDING ARTIFICIAL NUTRITION AND HYDRATION

In re Conroy

From 1983 to 1985 cases involving the withholding or withdrawing of artificial nutrition and hydration caused a great deal of discomfort and uncertainty. The first to bring the issue to national attention was a New Jersey case, *In re Conroy*.[9] Claire Conroy, a woman in her eighties, had organic brain syndrome and a host of other medical problems, including artheroschlerotic heart disease, hypertension, and diabetes. She eventually reached a point where she could not speak or even swallow sufficient amounts of nutrients to sustain herself, and a nasogastric feeding tube was inserted. She remained in a semifetal position and was unable to respond to verbal stimuli. In the opinion of her physician, she "probably had no higher function or consciousness." Still, she was not brain dead, comatose, or in a persistent vegetative state. Her legal guardian argued that she would never have permitted the insertion of the nasogastric tube in the first place. The facility was concerned and sought guidance from the court, which agreed with the surrogate's decision. However, the state's ombudsman intervened, saying that the failure to provide or the discontinuance of artificial nutrition and hydration would be construed as an act of homicide. Thus, this woman who had not seen a doctor in over 80 years now became prisoner to an unwanted device she never requested.

Meanwhile, in California, a 55-year-old patient who underwent a simple ostomy repair suffered severe anoxic depression in the recovery room. The chain of events included short staffing, nurse-physician conflict, ignoring of legal counsel advice, and spurious data. The decision[10] had a national impact and offered interesting guidance on how these kinds of situations should be handled.

The court argued that each pulsation of a ventilator and each drip of an IV feeding tube is equivalent to a manually administered dose. The court said that a respirator is really no more than a mechanical ambu bag. An ambu bag works by squeezing its contents out, then refills, then squeezes its contents out, then refills, and so forth. Similarly, an IV can be considered a substitute for a syringe. When someone depresses the plunger of a syringe, its contents are pushed out. During this process, the person is doing something—performing an act. After depletion, the person is not performing an act. If the person was to then insert a second syringe and push the plunger, that would be a whole other act. Accordingly, while the IV is dripping, an *act* is being performed. In between the drips, nothing is being done.

The court said that between the drips and pulsations there was no act involved and thus the failure to continue respiration or IV feeding or hydration was an *omission* consistent with good medical care. It could just have easily said the opposite, which is what the New Jersey courts initially maintained. Yet in the end the New Jersey Supreme Court, in the *Conroy* decision, adopted the same logic of California, and many other states followed suit.

Interestingly, the manner in which the *Barber* court determined that discontinuance of respiration or IV feeding or hydration was *acceptable medical practice* rather than *homicide* illustrates the incongruity between clinical and legal ways of establishing criteria for making decisions. This incongruity is reason enough to try to avoid going to court for a decision.

Cruzan v. Director, Missouri Department of Health

Cruzan[11] was a deviation from the legal legacy. Most cases had been based on the right of privacy, specifically the right to determine what happens to one's own body. In *Cruzan*, the focus was on the right to liberty instead of self-determination. The court also demanded a higher level of evidence than in previous cases. The standard shifted from "beyond a reasonable doubt," "a reasonable indication of patient intent," or "what the patient would likely have decided were he able to decide for himself" to "clear and convincing evidence standard." For example, even though the testimony of her family and her roommate showed that Nancy Cruzan had clearly indicated her wishes not to be kept alive when the circumstances were futile or hopeless, the court wanted more convincing material. The case was filled with legal gymnastics, and many briefs were filed on the part of Cruzan by national health care organizations. Among these was an excellent brief written on behalf of the American Hospital Association. It emphasized the historical right of the American family to make end-of-life decisions. Those who know the patient best should be given decision-making responsibility when that person is incapacitated from making decisions him- or herself.

In re Rosebush

A few years ago I was asked by the head of the Ethics and Humanities Division of the American Academy of Neurology to assist the attorneys arguing a case dealing with a young girl who, while waiting for a school bus, was hit by a pickup truck and seriously injured.[12] Her family exhausted every reasonable avenue of help, but after a year without a glimmer of hope they felt it was time for God to take her back, as they put it. The family was challenged by the facility in which their daughter resided, partly because it was receiving substantial reimbursement from the auto insurance company.

This case did not have the national impact that the other cases discussed did, but it is noteworthy for two reasons. First, Rosebush had a partially severed spinal cord and required a respirator to live; without it she would surely die. Second, the trial was a tremendous ordeal for the family. Day after day, the attorneys and the court berated the young girl's parents and grandparents. It was one of the most horrible things I have ever experienced. The family finally prevailed and were legally entitled to have the ventilator removed. Just as they heaved a sigh of relief, the prosecutor told them he would appeal the decision.

In re Michael Martin

A recent case, filed in Michigan, attempted to revive an effort to raise the level of proof required before a surrogate decision-maker, advocating on behalf of an incapacitated patient, could ask that life-prolonging medical procedures be discontinued. The Martin case[13] involved a patient who was neither terminally ill nor in a persistent vegetative state. His wife had been appointed his guardian and conservator.

In 1992, Michael Martin's wife requested that his artificially and technologically supplied nutrition be withdrawn. The hospital ethics committee determined that withdrawal was both ethically and medically appropriate, but that the hospital could not carry out the request without prior court approval. Mrs. Martin petitioned the court for the authorization to remove all nutritional support from her husband. Her husband's sister and mother filed an opposing petition.

Testimony given revealed that Michael Martin had indicated he would "rather die" than be dependent on someone for his care or be kept alive on a respirator. Even his sister testified that Michael had told her he did not want to be kept alive under those circumstances. The court determined that Michael Martin had not indicated "the exact circumstances" under which he would make such a choice. There were obviously strong dissenting opinions. This case is a vivid example of the importance of leaving well enough alone and proved to be a useless exercise of legal gymnastics that disenfranchised rather than supported patient self-determination.

SUMMARIZING THE LEGAL LEGACY

In *Quinlan*, the fundamental pivotal criterion on which decision should be based, was medical prognosis, which was decided by an "ethics" committee. If the patient could not be returned to a cognitive and sapient state, then life supports could be removed. The ethics committee's sole role in Quinlan was to determine whether her medical prognosis was indeed hopeless. The court noted that "the duty to treat diminishes as prognosis dims and when the prognosis is that of hopelessness, there is no need to continue *extraordinary treatment*." The court also felt that to become routinely involved in such matters would "constitute a gratuitous encroachment upon the medical profession."

In *Saikewicz*, the court argued that substituted judgment was the primary criterion for decision making. The substitute decision maker acts as if he or she were the person in whose behalf the decision is being made. The decision maker must take into account everything that has a bearing on the decision.

Dinnerstein clarified the criterion of substituted judgment and established that a DNR order can be charted in advance. In *Spring*, the court set forth 13 criteria for decision making and attempted to redefine the court's role. However, clinicians remained unclear about what weights would be assigned to the various components.

In re Eichner five criteria were established but then overridden by the New York Court of Appeals, which argued that it was unreasonable to demand such a cumbersome process be gone through. Interestingly, when the *Eichner v. Dillon* decision was handed down, it was heralded as the best example of how these cases ought to be decided. Of course, it is critical to examine the criteria upon which decisions were made prior to *Quinlan*, for perhaps *Eichner* was not a giant step forward but only a return to more sensible ways of resolving end-of-life issues.

Most would argue that prior to 1976 such decisions were basically made jointly by the doctor and the patient on the basis of some reasonable indication of patient intent. In other words, it seems as if care providers ventured through a thicket of legal ambiguity from 1976 to 1981, with all the attendant agony and grief, only to end up with the same standards they began with. In fairness, caregivers do have a richer understanding of the criteria involved in decision making for incompetent patients, but the price was great. The standards for decision making specifically for malpractice, however, did not change. The fundamental responsibility of the physician was and still is to act in accordance with the standards of the profession tempered by the wishes of the patient. During this period of legal clarification, the President's Commission on Ethical Issues in Biomedicine and Biomedical and Behavioral Research used insights gained from these cases to develop guidelines on decisions to forgo life support. See, for example, its helpful publication *Deciding to Forego Life Supports*, especially the chapter "The Elements of Decision Making." And in 1986, the AMA gave further clarification on withholding or withdrawing life-prolonging medical procedures which was further refined in 1994.[1]

The following ingredients are common to the kind of legal cases discussed above:

- a prognosis of hopelessness
- a reasonable indication of patient intent or a substituted judgment

- the question whether court permission should be sought or is required to withdraw or withhold treatment
- the question whether the physician has the authority to write an appropriate order in the patient's chart.

In situations of uncertainty, incorporating these key ingredients into the planning process gives some direction to decision making.

CONCLUSION

The legal legacy surrounding the protection of patient wishes is tortuous. Court decisions range from overintrusive paternalism to benign neglect. The clear implication of this review is that patient wishes regarding end-of-life issues need to be ascertained as early in the treatment process as possible (preferably even before treatment is necessary) and that when patient wishes are not ascertainable a mechanism must be in place to begin the process of determining what the patient would have wanted. This process cannot be effectively carried out under the pressure of crisis but must grow out of an understanding of the various roles that clinicians, the family, and, as a last resort, the courts should play. A sound knowledge of the legal concepts and realistic clinical alternatives that underpin decision making in this area is critical. Only with such knowledge will caregivers be able to act with confidence in providing medical treatment while at the same time protecting, not disenfranchising, the patient.

CASE STUDIES

Case 1

D. is HIV positive, and though he has been in a stable relationship with B., his girlfriend, he went to a crack house and wound up having sex with another woman. He contracted the virus either from this woman or from using a syringe to inject drugs. The nurse feels that B., who is pregnant, should be tested. D. has been encouraged to talk with B. but has not done so. An ethics consultant accompanies the attending physician to a meeting with D., his mother, and his girlfriend. The attending asks D., "Did you do what you told us you were going to do today?" The mother responds, "He sure did. What were you thinking about to get involved with a woman like that and bring this disease home?"

- Should the opportunity for counseling presented by this situation be passed up?
- Does the patient need to give permission for such a discussion? Or does confidentiality prevent this from happening?
- How does confidentiality relate to the protection of known innocent third parties?

Case 2

Mrs. B. is seriously ill. She has been successfully resuscitated three times in the past seven days. Prior to her admission to the hospital she was in a long-term care facility and had a chance to talk about her wishes regarding end-of-life issues. She has two sons, whom she characterizes as "screw-ups" with potential. Her impending death, partly because she will no longer be there to help direct their lives along the right path, is devastating to her. When approached about a "no-code" order she says that normally she would agree to a no-code but she feels she needs to show her sons that it is possible to fight to the end and wants to be coded.

- How does a discussion of medical futility affect her decision?
- Can or should clinical pathways or practice protocols and guidelines override the patient's wish?
- What could the caregivers do to help the patient help her sons so that she would not feel she had to undergo a course of futile treatment?
- What role should last wishes play in a case like this?
- Can the caregivers afford to honor the patient's wish?

Case 3

This scenario begins when the wishes of a patient or his surrogate cannot be clearly articulated. In an attempt to help stimulate the process of decision making, the doctor tells the family what he would do if it were his dad, the nurse offers an explanation of what her personal values are, the hospital administrator describes the total mission of the hospital, family members tell what they want, but no one knows what the patient wants.

- How best can the caregivers discover what the patient wants?
- What if the patient is incompetent? Are there other ways to identify patient wishes?
- How can the Saikewicz substituted judgment criterion assist the caregivers?
- By what standards should the caregivers be identifying patients' wishes?

Case 4

Mr. S. is severely dehydrated but is very afraid of "being another Karen Ann Quinlan" and wants no procedure or technology that he perceives to be an extraordinary measure, including use of an IV. His underlying medical condition is not terribly serious and he posesses decisional capacity but doesn't really seem to understand the implications of his refusal. The situation then arises that the caregivers disagree and feel his decision is wrong. The nurse is aware that Mr. S. is extremely opinionated, and she believes he could not possibly understand the implications of his refusal of an IV. "No sane person would make such a choice."

- What could the caregiver do in such a circumstance?
- Is this a conflict resolution issue?
- Is guardianship appropriate?
- Is surrogate decision making appropriate?

REFERENCES

1. Decisions Near the End of Life. *Chicago, American Medical Association Report.* 1991; 33(2).
2. *Schloendorff v. Society of New York Hospital*, 211 N.Y. 125, 105 N.E. 92 (1914).
3. *In re Quinlan*, 70 N.J. 10, 355 A.2d 647 (1976).
4. *Superintendent of Belchertown State School v. Saikewicz*, 370 N.E. 417 (1977).

Notes

5. *In re Dinnerstein*, 6 Mass. App. 380 N.E. 2d 134 (1978).

6. *In re Spring*, 380 Mass. 629, 405 N.E. 2d 115 (1980).

7. *In re Eichner*, 102 Misc. 2d 184, 423 N.Y. S. 2d 580 (N.Y. Sup. Dec. 6, 1979).

8. *Eichner v. Dillon*, 73 A.D. 2d 431, 426 N.Y.S. 2d 517 (N.Y.A.D. 2 Dept., Mar. 27, 1980), order modified by Storar, 52 N.Y. 2d 363, 420 N.E. 2d. 64, 438 N.Y.S. 2d 266 (N.Y., Mar. 31, 1981).

9. *In re Conroy*, 98 N.J. 321, 486 A. 2d 1209 (1983).

10. *Barber v. Superior Court*, 147 Cal. App. 3d 1006, 195 Cal. Rptr. 484 (Cal. Ct. App. 2d Dist. 1983).

11. *Cruzan v. Director, Missouri Department of Health*, 110 S. Ct. 2841 (1990).

12. *In re Rosebush*, No. 88-349180 AZ (Mich. Cir. Ct. Oakland County, July 29, 1988).

13. *In re Michael Martin*, 538 N.W. 2d 399 (Mich. Aug. 1995).

6

Formal Vehicles for Decision Making

ADVANCE DIRECTIVES

An advance directive is exactly what it says it is. It is a *directive* (written or otherwise expressed) *in advance* indicating what one would want or not want done in certain circumstances. Advance directives do not have to be written. They are often just verbal instructions given to physicians or other caregivers that are charted and honored. An advance directive may also be an earlier discussion or the significant content of a discussion or several discussions with family members, clergy, or friends. The word *directive* comes from the first living will statute in the United States, the California Natural Death Act. A living will was called a "directive to physicians," and the act stated that the physicians *must* act in accordance with the directive. Other states waffled on this issue and used the word *may* to relieve anxieties on the part of noncompliant physicians. California was the first state to take this step. California was also the first state to use and formally extend the durable power of attorney for medical decision making.

LIVING WILLS

A plethora of living wills have entered the health care arena in the past several years. This is somewhat odd because many states that have living will statutes have found them notoriously ineffective in ensuring patient wishes are honored and have typically adopted additional laws in a vain attempt to provide legislative certainty. A short investigation into these various legislative efforts to clarify end-of-life decisions will demonstrate the difficulties that a legislative solution often poses.

A living will is a written declaration or directive to physicians in which the patient ("declarant") affirms his or her wish not to be maintained by extraordinary means if he or she is terminally ill and if death is imminent. Imminence is defined in various ways. Maine offers the guideline "within a very short time," but within six months is the rule used in many other jurisdictions. A living will tries to anticipate a health care crisis and to prescribe a decision ahead of time. All living will acts require the following:

- The declarant must be found of sound mind when the living will is executed.
- The declarant must be terminally ill before the will takes effect.
- The declarant's death must be imminent when the will takes effect.
- Extraordinary measures will not be undertaken if they serve only to prolong life when the prognosis is hopeless. (Many state laws, oddly enough, exclude artificially supplied nutrition and hydration from the scope of extraordinary measures.)

Patients may create or customize their own living wills as well. If the patient has the foresight to execute a living will when competent and is able to affirm his or her intentions, the will can indeed be helpful. In the absence of the patient's later ability to interpret the declaration, however, clinicians and administrations may experience sufficient uncertainty about what the patient understood by the terms *imminent* and *extraordinary* that they refuse to honor the living will. Also, a patient may wish to refuse treatment even though he or she is not terminally ill and death is not imminent. A living will is often no help in these kinds of cases.

DURABLE POWER OF ATTORNEY

In an effort to further support the patient's right to determine his or her medical care in advance of a medical crisis, most states have chosen to supplement the living will with the durable power of attorney for medical decision making.

Originally, the durable power of attorney was designed to address specific problems associated with wills and estates. It was quickly recognized, however, that it was an excellent mechanism to help patients, clinicians, and administrators deal with some of the thornier problems of medical decision making. A power of attorney has long been recognized as a valid way to appoint someone else (an "agent") to act in the place of the person making the power (the "principal"). In common law, however, a power of attorney made by a competent adult was no longer effective if the principal became incompetent. The only solution was to follow the often time-consuming, complex, and expensive procedure of asking a court to appoint a guardian. Since guardianship was unnecessarily cumbersome in life-threatening situations, an easier mechanism to ensure respect for the patient's wishes was needed. Through a change in the law, a power of attorney was deemed to be "durable" (i.e., it would survive the disability or incapacity of the principal).

A durable power of attorney offers much greater breadth and flexibility than does a living will. The patient does not have to be terminally ill and facing imminent death but only temporarily incapacitated in order for the agent to exercise judgment, and the instrument can be used to ensure patient wishes are honored for a variety of choices surrounding specific health care procedures and therapeutic options. In terms of acceptance in the health care community, durable powers of attorney are "already on the books," and most states have specifically extended them to medical decision making under the title of "durable power of attorney for health care."

A willingness on the part of caregivers to accept a durable power of attorney for medical decision making can arise for a number of reasons. Some caregivers believe any reasonable indication of patient intent will suffice and that the information in a living will or a document appointing an agent virtually ensures the patient's wishes will be honored. Others are motivated by the fear of legal liability. For them, a legislatively authorized durable power of attorney for health care makes medical decision making much less complex and less uncertain and thereby reduces their discomfort.

Executing a durable power of attorney usually requires simply signing a document and (in some states) getting it notarized. No cumbersome guardianship proceedings need arise when the durable agent acts for the incapacitated principal. In most states, a durable power does not even have to follow a specific format, and durable powers executed in other states are generally considered valid.

It is important to recognize that durable powers of attorney are not right-to-die instruments. Rather, they are intended to ensure patient self-determination, and the outcome in a given instance could just as well be consent to treatment as refusal of treatment. One major objective is to avoid an emotionally charged confrontation between caregivers in the absence of the direct expression of wishes by the patient.

As already mentioned, a durable power of attorney survives the onset of incompetence. Appointing an agent under a durable power of attorney is a simple, inexpensive means of ensuring that the individual's wishes regarding choice of physician, use of intrusive procedures, and use of extraordinary life-prolonging measures are honored should the individual be unable to communicate them because of illness or senility.

A subtle yet important concern arises here. The durable agent is not a stranger appointed by a court, not a neutral or impartial spectator, but someone whom the patient, while competent, specifically designates to act for him or her in the event of an incapacitating illness or event. The appointment of someone who the patient trusts is much more in tune with the clinical perspective than is the use of a neutral court-appointed decision maker. In clinical environments, caregivers seek those who can best represent the patient's wishes or intent. In other words, they seek out and nurture partiality and shun impartial involvement.

Mark Fowler, in a *Columbia Law Review* article, captures the advantages of a durable power of attorney:

> From the patient's viewpoint, an agent would help to assure that an incapacitated patient receives treatment in accordance with his own wishes. Also, the appointment of an agent, unlike a living will, is respected. The agent could ask questions, assess risks and costs, speak to friends and relatives of the patient, consider a variety of therapeutic options, ask the opinion of other physicians, evaluate the patient's condition and prospects for recovery, in short, engage in the same complex decision-making process that the patient would undertake if he were

> able. . . . Thus, an agent extends the scope of the pa-
> tient farther than a written directive by making de-
> cisions consistent with the patient's values in situa-
> tions which he might not have specifically foreseen.
> Some basis for determining and documenting pa-
> tient intent even in the absence of an appointed
> agent is important.[1]

It is increasingly important to document the patient's wishes on the chart. If the patient has a living will, it still serves as a reasonable indication of patient intent and should be attached to the chart.

> An agent would provide someone to enforce the
> patient's treatment preferences, as well as permit
> the patient to appoint someone he trusts to repre-
> sent his interests. Unlike a living will, an agent is
> someone who is empowered to make decisions.[1]

The durable agent is someone with whom caregivers can talk and gain clarification as well as answers to his or her questions. If the clinician is unsure about the patient's wishes and there are no surrogates that can be identified to indicate what a person may have specifically meant in his living will, the clinician can hardly dissolve his uncertainty by talking to the living will document. A durable power of attorney will most of the time be a much better vehicle than anything that is written. Videotaping of patients articulating their wishes and choices can be helpful but does not replace the agent who can deal with issues that were unanticipated or unexpected.

The durable power of attorney is a wonderful mechanism for identifying patient wishes. A patient with serious head and neck cancer and a hopeless prognosis, while being video-taped for a teaching film on how to inform people they are dying, was asked "Do you want us to pound on your chest and stick a tube into you, and to have to go through a range of therapeutic furor?" He covered his tracheostomy site and re-sponded, "Well, they did that to me before and it saved my life, sure!" It is not part of the caregiving role to second-guess patients when they can tell us what they want. If they are able to express themselves, let them state what they want; if they are unable to do so, consulting an appointed agent is the best way to go.

SURROGACY LAWS

While the durable power of attorney has solved many problems, it is only effective if the agent is present. It is not uncommon for an elderly patient to appoint an agent the same age or older or a relative who lives in another state. As a result, when a medical crisis arises, the agent may not be present or may have since become incompetent. And, of course, many patients have not executed either a living will or a durable power of attorney for health care. Consequently, many state legislatures have enacted surrogate decision maker laws. These statutes provide that when an individual is determined to lack decisional capacity, the attending physician will identify a surrogate decision maker.

The surrogate decision maker is usually selected from the following candidates, which are listed in order of priority:

- durable medical agent
- anyone other than the durable agent specifically designated by the patient
- guardian of the person
- spouse
- parent
- adult child
- adult sibling
- adult grandchild
- close friend
- guardian of the estate

If there is a disagreement among members of the class of candidates (e.g., the adult children), a majority controls. If a majority cannot be determined, conflict resolution mechanisms may be instituted. If they cannot resolve the conflict, then a guardianship of the person is to be sought. A surrogate can act on behalf of the patient, like a durable agent, but the surrogate can only make decisions when the patient has a terminal illness and death is imminent and only with respect to life-prolonging medical treatment. Thus, the surrogate is relegated to acting in the same limited situations that are covered by a living will. Although the legislative approach has extended the range of decision makers, it still has not dealt with everyday medical treatment issues. An effective durable power of attorney is currently the only means to effectively resolve these issues.

PROBLEMS WITH ADVANCE DIRECTIVES

Patients do not have to be terminally ill to have their rights or wishes honored. Even patients who are terminally ill, however, may actually undermine their rights if they have executed an advance directive in certain states. In some cases, by executing a statutory living will or statutory-form health care surrogate designation, people may compromise their wishes more than if they had nothing. State-designed living will forms are often the result of political compromise. In the process of getting adopted they get watered down. They may compromise the patient who thinks he or she is getting something and may actually be giving something up that seemed innocuous at first glance, and it is unlikely that people signing the forms have read the statutes. Yet it is critical to know what restrictions such statutes impose. There are additional uncertainties as to what information must be collected, what must be asked of and told to patients, and how caregivers are to coordinate information regarding advance directives and pass it on from the hospital to the nursing home and from the nursing home to the hospice or home health care provider. Continuity of consent will likely become a major concern in the future.

Since these directives may compromise the wishes of patients, caregivers must be aware of this and warn patients about any restrictions such directives may impose. This is not meant to suggest that all statutory forms are bad. In fact, some are excellent. The point is that caregivers need to evaluate these forms carefully and see if they say what the patients or surrogates think that they say. If they do not, they will have to be amended. Let us examine the living will to see what problems it might present. A living will generally requires that three conditions be satisfied: the person whose will it is must be terminally ill, death must be imminent, and the person does not want extraordinary life-prolonging measures.

Imagine a physician who is uncomfortable and not sure what to do in an end-of-life situation. She consults an attorney who is relatively inexperienced in dealing with such matters and who looks to the living will statute for guidance. The attorney tells the physician that the statute precludes the removal of artificial nutrition and hydration. What should the physician do? Hopefully, the physician will act on the basis of what the patient wants and will properly upgrade and amend the patient's wishes via the chart. In the past, all a patient had to do was to tell his or her physician or surrogate of any change of mind and this information would have been written in the chart. The fact that patients now take the extra step of preparing a written document should afford them a greater degree of self-determination.

When procedures that are inconsistent with the wishes of the patient and do no more than prolong the dying process are imposed upon the patient, this is wrong. When medication and predigested, premeasured chemically created and prepared nutrition are injected into the patient through the nose or by means of a tube into the stomach against the wishes of the patient, this is wrong. Think of a patient who is in intractable pain and wants to die but whose life is being prolonged only because of a restriction in the living will statute. Feeding tubes should not have more rights than patients!

Caregivers can help avoid these situations by telling their patients about the limitations of these documents and by talking to them about their wishes. They can also inform their patients of the need to modify or replace these documents. In cases where a doctor has developed a relationship with a patient over the years, the problems with living wills can be dealt with relatively easily. In health care settings where little might be known about patients presenting with medical conditions, having advance directives or identifying a spokesperson is more important. Remember, advance directives were put into place because patients' wishes were not being honored by some doctors (who were creating unwanted and costly outliers). Those who already were comfortable honoring the wishes of their patients were not the problem.

The durable power of attorney for health care gives rise to few problems. It does not possess the same restrictions as the other advance directive options. Well-designed documents can help to ensure patient wishes are honored, resolve interfamilial decision-making conflict, and provide clear direction to hospitals and physicians.

A durable agent can both guard against and adjudicate conflict that arises in the clinical environment between family members who are split over what to do and can inform clinicians what the patient would have wanted. If a durable agent has not been appointed, caregivers should go out of their way to determine patient intent and then document it on the chart. This provides excellent insulation against potential liability and retains decision-making authority within the institution. It is obviously much easier for clinicians to talk and reason with an agent than talk with a written declaration. As already noted, one problem that can occur is the unavailability of the appointed durable agent at the point he or she is finally needed. Another is that the agent may be only marginally competent or, for whatever reason, may not be acting in the best interests of the patient.

LAG BETWEEN IDENTIFICATION OF ADVANCE DIRECTIVES AND ORDERS TO COMPLY

In working with diverse kinds of facilities, I have discovered there is often a lag between the identification of or the gaining of access to an advance directive and the actual writing of orders consistent with it. In the case of an advance directive indicating the requirement of writing an order to withhold cardiac and pulmonary resuscitation, it is important that the person who is primarily responsible for the patient's care be advised that there is such an advance directive. Suppose an order is not yet written but the nurse is aware there is an advance directive and knows what it states, should he or she honor the patient's wishes and refrain from resuscitation? As acuity increases, this and related problems will become more common, and health care policies will need to be altered to reflect the increase and its attendant problems.

TELEPHONE DNR ORDERS

A similar circumstance involves telephone do not resuscitate (DNR) orders. It is not uncommon for family members to take time before coming to terms with a DNR order. Imagine a brother and sister confronting the issue of whether to forego life-prolonging measures for their mother. They decide to tell the doctor to write a DNR order but they can't reach him immediately. In the meantime they tell the nurse responsible for their mother's nursing care about their decision. Before an order is written, the mother codes. This type of situation shows how important it is for caregivers to act on the basis of a reasonable indication of patient intent and develop appropriate policies and procedures.

POLICIES REGARDING ADVANCE DIRECTIVES

Occasionally family members ask or demand caregivers to do something that is medically inappropriate. They do this not because they do not care about their loved one, but because they have been misled or misinformed. A tired staff doctor may ask a patient's spouse, "Do you want us to *do everything*?" Doing everything is not a real option. Caregivers never do everything and they also never do absolutely nothing. Therefore, they must use language that is clinically appropriate rather than ask general questions that are inconsistent with medical standards.

Faced with uncertainty, caregivers feel they must do something, partly out of fear of legal liability. It is strange that they are often motivated by fear of legal liability and at the same time are unclear about how to insulate against legal liability. Even more lawyers who counsel health care facilities are often ill informed and have minimal training in health law. Many problems might be discovered to have simple solutions once health care professionals' legal duties are better understood.

The fear of legal liability stems mostly from the perceived risk of a negligence or malpractice suit. Remember that a negligence suit will be successful only if a duty was owed, there was a failure to act in accordance with that duty, there was an injury as a result of the breach, and the failure to act was the proximate cause of the injury. If caregivers want to insulate against legal liability, they need to show, i.e., by charting any advance directives, that they fulfilled their duty not to "do everything."

Unfortunately, caregivers are not always entirely sure how to articulate or explain what their duty is. If they are unclear about their duty, they obviously will not be able to show they fulfilled their duty. When asked what their duty is, caregivers usually say it is to "do no harm." Although true, this is too general an answer. They must be able to explain in detail what constitutes appropriate medical care in the situation in question. Hopefully, as practice guidelines, practice parameters, and clinical pathways are created, some of the confusion in knowing what to do will be minimized.

THE IMPORTANCE OF CREATING SENSIBLE POLICIES

As mentioned, caregivers have a duty to act in accordance with the standards of the medical profession. The best way to *demonstrate* that they have fulfilled their duty is through ongoing documentation. In addition, they must develop policies that give direction in end-of-life cases and provide education about standards and major legal decisions. Refining their communication skills will certainly help as well. They must be able, for example, to describe realistic medical alternatives to surrogate decision makers. In many cases, patients and surrogates say they want everything to be done because caregivers ask the wrong questions in the wrong way at the wrong time. Patients and surrogates need adequate support and guidance.

It is often helpful to crystallize the best way to approach a type of problem by creating a policy. For example, a policy on withholding and withdrawing life-prolonging medical procedures is extremely important. It can better assure the wishes of the patient as well as better insulate the hospital and clinicians from potential legal liability. Having a policy in place, however, is not enough. Appropriate in-service education to make those who use the policy comfortable with it is critical. The education and policy development process also involves educating the in-house attorney about medical procedures used in end-of-life cases so that he or she can become more helpful and provide advice on documentation.

A policy on informed consent should ensure that consent is not mere acquiescence but reflects the patient's wishes. Ideally, the consent process should result in the patient's honest consent to clinically realistic treatments and alternatives. Learning from the mistakes and successes of others rather than having to remake the mistakes is the best strategy. Clinical education has to provide a better understanding of caregivers' legal obligations and the importance of documentation for demonstrating the fulfillment of these obligations. Effective and timely communication with patients and their families should be the rule rather than the exception. By honestly sharing medical realities, caregivers can help patients form reasonable desires and make sensible decisions.

By attempting extensive life-prolonging measures to avoid the risk of liability, caregivers will often exacerbate their problems. Practicing good medicine, providing good nursing care, making appropriate referrals, and demonstrating that the patient has given truly informed consent are the best protections.

Informed consent, both as an indicator of patient wishes and as an insulator against legal liability, is an essential foundation of policies regarding the withholding and withdrawing of life-prolonging medical treatment. If informed consent plays the role it should, a DNR order, for example, then becomes merely an order generated by virtue of a well-grounded patient wish. Indeed, informed consent is one of the most important means available for dealing with end-of-life issues as well as ensuring against potential legal liability.

DOCUMENTING CONTROVERSY

The way in which caregivers document ethical problems that arise is of extreme importance, particularly when there is disagreement among parties, be they clinicians or family members. The best advice is to document controversy in an ongoing and dynamic way that is consistent with good clinical care. To explain this more clearly, I will describe a concrete example. Imagine a patient who has chronic obstructive pulmonary disease and indicates clearly that should he suffer cardiac or pulmonary arrest he does not want to be resuscitated. He has been resuscitated before and now believes that it is his time to die. His doctor talks about the implications of this decision. She tells the patient that she understands that he does not want to be a prisoner to a machine but that there are acutely reversible episodes that she can get him through by means of effective and well-proven medical procedures. The patient says that he knows he has the right to refuse treatment and that he has suffered enough. He trusts his caregivers but is concerned that his family will try to override his wishes when he no longer possesses the capacity to speak for himself.

The doctor suggests a durable power of attorney be established for the patient. The patient says he does not know anyone on whom he can rely. Besides, he and the doctor have discussed this issue several times and the doctor knows what he wants. The doctor is concerned about how she should document the patient's desire for a DNR order to be written.

The nurse who has been at the bedside during this discussion thinks that having the DNR order written is important. She feels that the amount of time that she has spent with the patient (much more time than the doctor has spent) has allowed her to get to know the patient much better than the doctor does. She has been documenting in the nursing notes what the patient has said, but she thinks the doctor needs to do something as well. What she is really uncomfortable about is that the doctor has not made notes about the patient's fears and the potential controversy that will likely arise. She remembers what happened to other patients in the past, and she thinks it is critically important to document the controversy and even include the specific words the patient used.

Caring for people at the end of life includes allaying their fears that their wishes will not be honored and they will become prisoners of some technology. Since they may well lose decisional capacity, their caregivers must take special steps to protect their wishes by documenting them. If a family member is appointed guardian of a patient who is decisionally incapacitated, the doctor will become relatively helpless to honor the patient's wishes, short of some court action. Thus to ensure the wishes of the patient are honored and protect against the potential legal action by the family, the doctor must document not only that the patient does not want to be resuscitated but that the patient believes that when he is vulnerable and unable to protect his own interests his family will take advantage of his circumstance.

Institutional conflict resolution procedures can be used to protect patients, caregivers, and the facility. In dealing with conflict, the clinician begins by talking with the family members and documenting the significant content of the discussion. The clinician may then call in a social worker or someone from pastoral care. Whatever staff becomes involved should document their interventions. Creating a paper trail that records the patient's wishes and shows the family is of a different mind is a necessary part of the consent process. If a guardian is sought when the patient becomes incapacitated, notes of the discussions can be used to ensure that the patient's wishes are not compromised. If the clinicians caring for the patient are concerned that family members are likely to become adversarial, they may want to call another clinician in to confirm the decisional capacity of the patient as a further precautionary measure. This makes it harder for a guardian to argue that the patient did not know what he or she was doing or did not understand what his or her decision meant. Referrals can be used to confirm consent just as they are used to confirm a medical diagnosis. Referring the case to the ethics committee can also serve as an important protection for the patient.

MATTERS OF CONSCIENCE

Many practice acts and some advance directive legislation include room for matters of conscience. Caregivers have a right to self-determination as well as patients, and thus they should not be forced to do what they feel is wrong and/or inconsistent with their religious or personal tenets. If indeed a matter of conscience creates a conflict between what the patient wants and what the caregiver is willing to do, the caregiver must inform the patient as well as identify another caregiver to replace him or her.

Claiming that reluctance to treat a patient is a matter of conscience can be a convenient way to avoid dealing with issues that are difficult or uncomfortable. When initial concerns about caring for AIDS patients arose, it was amazing to me how many caregivers "had difficulty" dealing with such patients. Legitimate refusals to treat based on conscience should be respected, but sorting out the legitimacy of refusals is important.

At the institutional level, matters of conscience are more problematic. Although an institution is obligated to identify up front any procedures it is unwilling to perform, its refusal to perform procedures has to be consistent with the state law as well as the constitutional rights of patients. The right of patients to make decisions about their care includes the right to change their minds as they get older and sicker. Must a patient go elsewhere if he or she has lived in a long-term care facility for many years but now has decided to ask not to be resuscitated, a request that is inconsistent with the "conscience of the facility?" The answer to this question is unclear. Having a policy in place that clarifies how such changes of mind will be dealt with can be helpful. It shows at the very least that the actions are not serendipitous but rather in accordance with established policies.

CASE STUDIES

Case 1

After two friends had died within the past two years, Mrs. D. grew concerned that her wish not to be kept alive on artificial nutrition and hydration might not be honored. She appointed a close friend about the same age to be her durable agent. Many years previously, she had filled out a living will form. Eventually Mrs. D.'s condition deteriorated and she no longer possessed the capacity to voice her wishes. Her durable agent was sought to act in her stead but this person had already died and the living will had expired.

- On what basis should decisions be made?
- What effect on decision making does an expired directive have?
- What might the caregiver do for direction?
- Should the facility's ethics committee be consulted? If so, what can it do?
- Suppose the living will had not expired but instead included a provision requiring that artificial nutrition and hydration not be withheld.

Case 2

Mr. J., who has Alzheimer's disease, has drafted an advance directive saying that if he was to suffer an infection that might be reversible with antibiotics, he wishes to refuse the antibiotics.

He does not want to deteriorate any more and believes that the septicemia that might result would be "an old man's friend."

- Should his wish be honored?
- Do you have to be terminally ill to exercise the right to refuse treatment?
- Can people with Alzheimer's still have the capacity to make medical decisions?

Case 3

N., while driving to Florida, is involved in a car accident in Georgia and is seriously injured. Attempts to treat her injuries have been somewhat successful but her condition remains critical and she may die. She has a living will from her home state of Kentucky that was found in her glove box.

- Should the facility honor the wishes expressed in her living will?
- Is the living will likely to be a sufficient indicator of what the patient would want to have done?
- How should the caregiver document the living will?
- Should an attempt to identify a surrogate or enlist other aids to decision making be undertaken?

REFERENCE

1. Fowler M. Appointing an agent to make medical treatment choices. *Columbia Law Review.* 84:985.

7

Developing Institutional Policies on Ethical Issues

Much has changed in the 20 years since the insights of the President's Commission established pursuant to the Quinlan decision were first publicized. Acute and postacute facilities alike are beginning to realize that the best way to deal with such issues as withholding/withdrawing mechanical ventilation and artificial nutrition and hydration is through the development of clear policies. What is emerging is that education and clarification have been insufficient to date. Policies and procedures are also required.

There are many reasons for the development of appropriate policies. For example, physicians and administrators assume that hospital lawyers will have clear answers to the questions that arise, but this is rarely the case. Many lawyers who work in health care settings are not trained in health care law and thus find they need on-the-job training. As a result, the advice offered is often excessively cautious. Accordingly, such attorneys are often perceived as "paid paranoids" operating in an unfamiliar milieu and are often more comfortable handling the legal tasks involved in administration than providing guidance in the making of treatment decisions.

Most of the problems caregivers face arise less from the complexity of the issues than from a reluctance to make decisions and a tendency to dump decision-making responsibility on others. Attending physicians, for example, often avoid decision making by funneling it to the hospital legal counsel, the ethics committee, the medical director, risk managers, or pastoral care workers. These other professionals, although well intentioned, may act as enablers and infantilize physicians. It is of course important to distinguish this process of discomfort and infantilization from the process of making a proper referral. I in no way mean to suggest that the individual caregiver who needs additional information or advice to make a decision should not seek that information or advice.

111

THE RISING IMPORTANCE OF ADMINISTRATIVE ETHICS

There is a renewed emphasis on addressing ethical issues in health care facilities and agencies. This has been stimulated by a variety of factors, not the least of which are the new Joint Commission guidelines for organizational ethics in home health and long-term care organizations. The guidelines concern such areas as the relationships that an organization has with other organizations and its mechanisms for conflict resolution. Complying with such mandates is an obviously important new incentive in postacute care.

Since the failure to comply with these mandates can be viewed now as a regulatory violation, the associated issues will receive even greater administrative scrutiny than in the recent past. Administrative support of an ethics program can set a positive tone for the organization.

Corporate or systemwide mission statements and principles provide direction as well. Policies are an excellent means of integrating promises made to patients and clinical and organizational commitments. They protect caregivers from liability by providing guidance and ensuring consistency. Also they can be appealed to where there is a crisis or challenge.

Supporting or sponsoring an ethics program sends a positive message to the staff and can dramatically shape the way in which staff members interact with and react to their patients and fellow staff members. Doing something because it is a good thing or the right thing to do has different implications than being forced to comply with a mandate. If staff see that administrators treat others well and honor their wishes, they may gain confidence that they will be treated right and may feel a greater allegiance to the organization.

Administrators can create an overall impression and set the stage for a positive response by the staff. Staff will assume ownership of a policy if they were involved in developing it and their concerns were voiced and taken into account. Creation of an ethics committee, identifying ethics resources, sharing insights, and identifying strengths and weaknesses to be addressed all can enhance an ethics program and policy development.

It does not make sense to develop excellent policies if the staff remains ignorant of what they are and why they were written and how they differ from previous policies. Policies such as the facility's integrated consent policy should be developed in concert with clinicians (so it has a sound clinical base) and be reviewed by the medical staff and quality assurance. Once this has been done, however, it becomes an administrative policy.

The creation of an administrative policy will give the administrator more authority to deal with issues that in the past may have been perceived as overstepping his or her bounds and stepping too far onto the clinical turf. When an administrative policy is not being followed and it is not merely a manner of clinical style or judgment that is at stake, it is appropriate for the administrator to intervene or for other caregivers to question an action or failure to act. This can have a positive effect on the facility's quality assurance and risk management profile.

THE PROCESS OF CONSENT

A wide range of ethical issues are encompassed by the general issue of consent and many of these issues, while distinctive, are closely related to each other. For example, the question of whether to withhold or withdraw artificially or technologically supplied respiration, nutrition, and hydration should not be decided independent of the patient's wishes.

It is important not only to understand what role patient wishes and informed consent play in the decision-making process but also to recognize that documenting this process is an important way to protect against legal liability. We are more effective at achieving this through acting in accordance, rather than discordance, with patient wishes or those of a designated surrogate when the patient is unable to express him- or herself.

Misunderstandings about Consent

Caregivers often misunderstand how they should deal with consent. I frequently ask clinicians involved in seminars to fill in the appropriate verb in the following sentence: "From the perspective of the caregiver, it is important to _____ consent." Consistently the word *obtain* is offered as the first and often the only choice. At the same time, some will say that the sentence needs to be changed. "What good is consent," they ask, unless it is "informed" consent? It is not just permission that caregivers require but permission from someone who possesses the capacity to understand and appreciate the significance of what is being said.

In any case, the verb *obtain* betrays a misunderstanding about consent. It suggests consent is indeed something that can be obtained once and for all as if it were no more than a legal transaction or discrete static event. Instead, consent should be viewed as a dynamic and ongoing process. Patients come into a facility near death and leave healthy or come in reasonably healthy and leave in a worsened condition or quite dead. Decision making changes as the clinical course changes, so having a static transaction makes little clinical or legal sense. Despite this, consent is frequently discussed not as a dynamic process but instead as a form of contract that exists between the doctor and the patient. This seems odd, for one of the fundamental requisites of a contract is that the parties be on equal footing. It seems strange to think that clinicians, with their wealth of experience and knowledge, can be perceived as being on equal footing with their patients. In addition, patients generally get all their information about prognosis, risks, benefits, and alternatives from caregivers. Patients put themselves in caregivers' hands; caregivers should support them. Policies can strengthen caregivers' hands rather than make them shake with trepidation in the face of uncertainty. It is the spirit of the activity, rather than the protocol, that dictates the reasonableness of the activity, and policies should set forth the tone and spirit of caregivers' perceptions about consent and their duties to those whom they serve.

The legal use of consent involves demanding the patient's signature on a consent form. From an ethical perspective, the consent process should be aimed at allowing the patient to become actively involved in his or her care. Caregivers should thus transmit information in a way that is intelligible and not demanding. The ethical stance of supporting and caring for patients arises from a sense of professional duty and a sense of the duty owed to all other human beings—to help them in contexts where they would otherwise be overwhelmed. The legal responsibility concerns the nature, adequacy, and intelligibility of the information as well as the alternatives that are provided and the explanations of potential risks that are offered. How can someone consent to something without knowing the range of options available to him or her?

Defensive medicine has to some extent contributed to caregivers seeing law as primary and ethics as secondary. After all, although attention to ethics may give caregivers more professional satisfaction, ethical problems do not often keep them awake in quite the same way as potential lawsuits. That does not, however, provide license to treat patient wishes lightly.

CONSENT AND DUTY

Once caregivers realize the importance of informed consent, both as an indicator of patient wishes and as an insulator against legal liability, they can better ensure that the wishes of patients are honored. From a legal perspective, the clearer it is that caregivers have fulfilled their duty to *cultivate* informed consent, the less exposure they will have to the risk of allegations of negligence. Acting in accordance with the wishes of the patients should be the foundation of policies regarding the withholding and withdrawing of life-prolonging medical procedures. A request for a do not resuscitate (DNR) order is merely an example of patient wish, that is, a wish not to be resuscitated should one go into cardiac arrest. These requests are not divorced from medical standards, for part of the information component is to talk about the appropriateness of interventions and probable outcomes.

Caregivers must protect patients from overtreatment as well as undertreatment. For example, suppose a patient is very sick and the prognosis is poor. The patient should be informed of what reasonable options exist. If she "wanted everything to be done," the caregiver would lay out what this might mean and try to get her to make a medically viable and reasonable choice. He might respond to her wanting everything to be done by saying, "Certainly we'll do everything that makes sense to keep you comfortable and we won't do things that do no more than cause you discomfort and prolong the dying process."

The guiding thread which holds the individual sections and concerns within the policy is consent. Consent is a critical component of the twofold duty that clinicians owe to their patients: to act in accordance with the standards of the profession and to act in accordance with the patients' wishes. It is unusual for a malpractice suit to be brought that does not include an allegation that consent was either improper, insufficient, or absent. As already noted, caregivers often mistakenly view consent as something that must be obtained—a piece of paper or a form that, once completed, is put into the chart and not worried about.

The model of "obtaining consent" is not consistent with the way medicine is practiced. Clinical care is dynamic, consent must be congruent with the clinical process, and so it must be dynamic as well.

Perhaps a short etymological excursion into consent will help us shift our focus of consent as something we obtain to that of a dynamic process more congruent with clinical care. Consent comes from two Latin words: *con* meaning "with" and *sentire* meaning both "to know" and "to feel."

Viewed in this way, consent requires continual transmission of information to the patient as circumstances change. The nature of this information as well as the manner in which it is shared or transmitted play a very important role in the decision-making process. What has to be afforded is information as to the risks and benefits of a suggested treatment and available alternatives. The information must be shared in a supportive way where the patient (or surrogate decision maker) is given regular opportunities to be involved in the process. Rather than obtaining consent, caregivers should "nurture" or "cultivate" consent. They must make certain that their patients understand all important information and that the patients feel the caregivers are making an honest attempt to understand and appreciate their wishes and to act in accordance with them. This does not mean that caregivers have to share information in a neutral way but only that they have to provide appropriate information in a supportive milieu.

INTEGRATED CONSENT POLICIES

As mentioned above, policies help ensure that the wishes of patients are respected while at the same time insulating the facility and clinicians against potential legal liability. Having good policies in place, however, is not enough. Appropriate in-service education to familiarize staff, including physicians and in-house attorneys, with the policies is critical.

Developing a policy which better assures informed consent not as acquiescence but as a reasonable indication of the patient's wishes is critical. It is better to develop policies before a crisis arises than to develop them as a tourniquet to staunch the bleeding. In my view, it is also better to integrate related policies into a single overarching policy. This avoids having to deal with a morass of divergent and often overlapping policies, such as DNR policies, artificial nutrition and hydration policies, emergency consent policies, and so on. In the case of an integrated policy, issuing a DNR order (more properly, an order to withhold cardiac or pulmonary resuscitation) is merely an instance of obeying the patient's wishes based on medical information regarding probable outcomes, risks, alternatives, and the like. The decision to withhold or withdraw other life-prolonging procedures would follow as a natural consequence of the DNR order. This is a separate decision, yet it would not be made without a DNR decision being made first.

In addition to ensuring patient autonomy and allowing physicians to perform without excessive fear, an integrated policy can be an excellent marketing tool and provide a means of addressing costly outliers that have been generated by physician discomfort and delays in decision making.

DEVELOPING AN INTEGRATED POLICY COMBINING BROAD CONSENT WITH WITHDRAWING/ WITHHOLDING LIFE-PROLONGING MEDICAL PROCEDURES ISSUES

An integrated policy dealing with broad consent as well as with withholding/withdrawing life-prolonging medical procedures should incorporate legal safeguards and ethical standards, conform to the constitutional rights of patients, and be clinically realistic. It must also be tailored to meet the needs of the particular institution.

The policy should offer guidance to clinicians and clarify the institution's commitment to the community it serves. The policy can serve as a marketing tool by showing the institution cares about patients and goes to some pains to ensure their wishes are honored.

It is important to set the tenor of the policy by beginning on a positive note. The first sentence might read something like this: "Your wishes play an important part in shaping your care."

A definition section can be added to minimize ambiguity and offer consistency and guidance. Three sample definitions follow:

- **informed consent.** The permission given by a patient (or surrogate) to allow a medical treatment to be performed after he or she has been reasonably counseled regarding his or her condition, the nature and purpose of proposed treatment, the probable risks, the prognosis, the expected probable outcomes, and the implications of foregoing treatment. The counseling should be done in such a way that the patient (or surrogate) understands and appreciates the significance of the information provided.
- **surrogate.** Someone who acts in the patient's stead (substitutes in judgment for the patient) to determine what the patient would likely have decided were he or she able to decide for him- or herself. Also, someone appointed through the surrogate act to act for the patient.
- **terminally ill.** A designation used to refer to those who suffer from terminal disease and whose prognosis is extremely poor. In most cases, death is imminent or the patient suffers from an ongoing deteriorative or degenerative disease, and further interventions are viewed as only prolonging the dying process.

Since confusion abounds regarding "who decides," the policy should include discussion of this issue. Although the body of the policy addresses consent for the patient who has the capacity to make decisions, clarification regarding surrogate or substitute decision making is necessary. Also, a DNR order does not entail withholding other life supports (e.g., artificial nutrition and hydration, antibiotics, blood, and antiseizure medications), but it does set the stage for discussing their withholding or withdrawal.

The integrated model recommended here has been adopted by facilities in several states, including California,

Virginia, New Jersey, Kentucky, Michigan, and West Virginia. It has benefited from the insight of physicians, nurses, social workers, administrators, and lawyers, and it offers a framework for clinicians, patients, and surrogate decision makers to use in dealing with a wide range of related issues.

Proper development and implementation of an integrated informed consent and withholding or withdrawal of life-prolonging procedure policy should be a top priority. The implementation process should include solid in-service education for the clinical staff.

An integrated policy "integrates" clinical and administrative ethics, is an excellent risk management tool, and creates a more stable working environment. It is an alternative to the constellation of disjointed policies that cause problems of inconsistency in many health care institutions. In an integrated policy, each section builds upon and at the same time reinforces the other sections, giving the policy internal strength and coherence.

A SAMPLE INTEGRATED POLICY

Introduction to the Provisions of the Policy

It is essential to ensure that the wishes of each patient be supported and respected. The initiation of many medical and nursing interventions require that permission be given by the patient or a surrogate (often a spouse or family member). This permission is referred to as consent. In order for the patient to make an informed choice, the attending physician is responsible for informing the patient or surrogate (when the patient is unable to participate in decision making by virtue of disability or incapacity) about the patient's condition, the nature and purpose of proposed treatment, the probable risks, the prognosis, and the expected probable outcomes. The imparting of the information should be done in such a way that the patient understands and appreciates the significance of what is being discussed and explained. If the patient has been adequately informed, the patient's permission is referred to as informed consent.

Consent is a legal privilege that allows one to do what in the absence of that consent would not be acceptable. It is an extension of an individual's right to privacy (often expressed as the right of self-determination) and in health care encompasses the right to have one's wishes honored so long as those wishes are consistent with the ethical integrity of the medical profession. It is the patient (or a designated surrogate if the patient's wishes are unknown or unclear) who consents and the patient's right of self-determination shall not be facilely compromised. Consent is not something one obtains, nor is it a static legal transaction; instead it is a process to be cultivated. Where decisional capacity fluctuates and it is unclear to the clinician whether the patient has the capacity to make a given decision, further assessment will be made. If the medical condition of the patient interferes with the patient's capacity to decide, then attempts will be made to correct the condition when possible to enable the patient to better participate in medical decision making.

There are times when a physician may want to administer life-saving medical therapy that is inconsistent with the wishes of a patient who is not terminally ill, in a chronic or persistent vegetative state, in the later stages of a deteriorative or degenerative disease process, or faced with a serious irreversible condition. In such circumstances, after adequate attempts to inform the patient of the reversibility of his or her condition, the physician must honor the wishes of the patient or surrogate decision maker. Adults with the capacity to make medical decisions have the right to determine what shall be done with their own bodies, and the patient shall not have wishes he or she expressed in advance (or his or her likely wishes as determined by a surrogate decision maker) thwarted or undermined.

If the patient, by virtue of disability or incapacity, is unable to express his or her wishes and there are no prior expressed wishes or advance directives, then another may serve as a surrogate for the patient and exercise "substituted judgment" on his or her behalf. The surrogate should attempt to determine what the patient's wishes were or what the patient would likely have decided were the patient able to decide for him- or herself.

Order of Priority of Decision Makers

It is mandated that nonhospital postacute settings have safeguards in place to ensure patient (or resident) autonomy.

Since patients in long-term care facilities often reside in these facilities for long periods of time, often many years, it is important that they be given the opportunity to make their wishes known. In home health, the absence of physicians during the provision of care is a significant factor as well, and home health patients need to be provided the same opportunity. This is particularly important where family members may disagree with the wishes of a competent patient. In such circumstances, the patient should be urged to identify someone to speak for him or her. The order of priority of decision makers is generally as follows: the durable medical agent, anyone specified by the patient, a legal guardian with specific authority to make medical decisions or decisions of person, the spouse, children of age, and parents.

Others may be sought to gain clarification or further indication of the patient's/resident's wishes (e.g., the patient's primary physician, clergy, and longstanding friends). If members of a specific class, such as children of age, disagree, some attempt to resolve the conflict consistent with the facility's conflict resolution policies should be made.

Advance directives, such as living wills, health care surrogate designations or durable powers of attorney, should be evaluated for appropriateness as extenders of the self-determination of the patient and should be integrated into the decision-making process in accordance with the spirit with which these formal tools were drafted. Copies of advance directives should be documented and placed in the patient's chart. The chart should also identify agents or surrogates and how they can be reached and integrated into the decision-making process.

Continuity of Consent

Patient wishes documented during former hospitalizations or treatment in other health care settings can often serve as a helpful guide for future decision making. Information about expressed wishes should be integrated into the decision-making process and upgraded and re-evaluated as indicated. It is particularly important for minimizing uncertainty and confusion when a patient experiences an acute medical episode and initiating or withholding life-prolonging medical treatment may pivot on the patient's prior directives. It can also serve as a safeguard of the patient's autonomy as he or she travels across the health care continuum.

Emergency Consent

When an emergency of sufficient magnitude warrants immediate action; the patient, by virtue of his or her physical or mental condition, is unable to consent to appropriate treatment; there are no prior wishes indicating that the treatment not be initiated; a designated surrogate is not available; and it is believed that the treatment will likely reverse an acutely reversible process, the treatment may be initiated. The goal in such circumstances is to stabilize the patient so that the immediate danger is removed. After the patient has been stabilized, his or her wishes regarding further treatment should be sought and honored in accordance with the spirit of the integrated informed consent policy. If the patient is unable to provide consent and a surrogate is not available, the nursing supervisor should be notified so he or she can institute procedures to locate the appropriate surrogate decision maker.

Orders Not To Resuscitate

There are times when a patient directly or indirectly (via a surrogate decision maker) will express the wish not to be resuscitated in situations where such resuscitation would serve only to prolong the patient's suffering or extend an otherwise futile course of treatment. Such a wish is not to be taken lightly. However, if the physician believes the condition is potentially reversible, then a significant attempt to inform the patient of this and persuade the patient to re-evaluate his or her decision is in order. The physician must explain the implications of this decision to the patient. If the patient is unmoved, the physician should write a DNR order—an order to withhold cardiac and/or pulmonary resuscitation. (An order to "do everything" or "do nothing" is meaningless and requires further clarification.)

It is important to recognize that the decision to withhold medical procedures must be an informed decision and must be congruent with the clinical process. Accordingly, it requires upgrading, refining, and re-evaluating as appropriate. There may be times when the DNR order may be temporarily suspended (e.g., during certain diagnostic procedures or during palliative surgery). If such an option is contemplated, it should be discussed with the patient and documented.

The attending physician should determine the appropriateness of a DNR order for any given medical condition based upon the prognosis and the patient's wishes. Once the DNR decision has been made, the attending physician should write a formal DNR order, document it in the progress notes, and evaluate its appropriateness periodically.

Withholding/Withdrawing Other Life-Prolonging Medical Procedures

The policy outlined here is consistent with the guidelines of the President's Commission for the Study of Ethical Problems in Medicine and Biomedical and Behavioral Research as well as the opinion of the American Medical Association's Council of Ethical and Judicial Affairs on Withholding or Withdrawing Sustaining Medical Treatment (Exhibit 7-1). The question of withholding or withdrawing life-prolonging procedures most often arises when the prognosis for recovery is extremely poor; when the patient is terminally ill, suffers from an ongoing deteriorative or degenerative disease, or is in a chronic and persistent vegetative state; or when further interventions are perceived as likely to merely prolong the dying process. After sufficient data have been obtained to confirm the patient's prognosis and wishes, then withdrawal or withholding of life-prolonging medical treatment may be initiated. Efforts to maintain patient comfort (e.g., mouth and skin care and symptom control) will continue.

Life-prolonging medical procedures include medication and artificially or technologically supplied respiration, nutrition, and hydration. Questions regarding care for patients who will not benefit from continued therapy but have unrealistic expectations are increasingly common. The dynamic process of informed consent should allow the patient or family members an opportunity to revise decisions as the prognosis changes. The physician is a critical player in this process.

Exhibit 7-1 Opinion of the AMA Council of Ethical and Judicial Affairs on Withholding or Withdrawing Sustaining Medical Treatment*

The social commitment of the physician is to sustain life and relieve suffering. Where the performance of one duty conflicts with the other, the preferences of the patient should prevail. The principle of patient autonomy requires that physicians respect the decision to forego life-sustaining treatment of a patient who possesses decisionmaking capacity. Life-sustaining treatment is any treatment that serves to prolong life without reversing the underlying medical condition. Life-sustaining treatment may include, but is not limited to, mechanical ventilation, renal dialysis, chemotherapy, antibiotics, and artificial nutrition and hydration.

There is no ethical distinction between withdrawing and withholding life-sustaining treatment.

A competent, adult patient may, in advance, formulate and provide a valid consent to the withholding or withdrawal of life-support systems in the event that injury or illness renders that individual incompetent to make such a decision.

If the patient receiving life-sustaining treatment is incompetent, a surrogate decisionmaker should be identified. Without an advance directive that designates a proxy, the patient's family should become the surrogate decisionmaker. Family includes persons with whom the patient is closely associated. In the case when there is no person closely associated with the patient, but there are persons who both care about the patient and have sufficient relevant knowledge of the patient, such persons may be appropriate surrogates. Physicians should provide all relevant medical information and explain to surrogate decisionmakers that decisions regarding withholding or withdrawing life-sustaining treatment should be based on substituted judgment (what the patient would have decided) when there is evidence of the patient's preferences and values. In making a substituted judgment, decisionmakers may consider the patient's advance directive (if any); the patient's values about life and the way it should be lived; and the patient's attitudes towards sickness, suffering, medical procedures, and death. If there is not adequate evidence of the incompetent patient's preferences and values, the decision should be based

continues

Exhibit 7-1 continued

on the best interests of the patient (what outcome would most likely promote the patient's well-being).

Though the surrogate's decision for the incompetent patient should almost always be accepted by the physician, there are four situations that may require either institutional or judicial review and/or intervention in the decisionmaking process: (1) there is no available family member willing to be the patient's surrogate decisionmaker, (2) there is a dispute among family members and there is no decisionmaker designated in an advance directive, (3) a health care provider believes that the family's decision is clearly not what the patient would have decided if competent, and (4) a health care provider believes that the decision is not a decision that could reasonably be judged to be in the patient's best interests. When there are disputes among family members or between family and health care providers, the use of ethics committees specifically designed to facilitate sound decisionmaking is recommended before resorting to the courts.

When a permanently unconscious patient was never competent or had not left any evidence of previous preferences or values, since there is no objective way to ascertain the best interests of the patient, the surrogate's decision should not be challenged as long as the decision is based on the decisionmaker's true concern for what would be best for the patient.

Physicians have an obligation to relieve pain and suffering and to promote the dignity and autonomy of dying patients in their care. This includes providing effective palliative treatment even though it may foreseeably hasten death.

Even if the patient is not terminally ill or permanently unconscious, it is not unethical to discontinue all means of life-sustaining medical treatment in accordance with a proper substituted judgment or best interests analysis.

*Code of Medical Ethics Current Opinions, with Annotations, 1994 edition, Chicago: American Medical Association, pgs. 36–37.

Note: The AMA Council on Ethical and Judicial Affairs is the judicial authority of the AMA. The primary function of the council is to establish ethics policy and perform judicial review. This opinion is the latest version of the council's work in this area which was originally created in 1981.

Such policies should be a conscious effort to create an architecture into which patients/residents can more comfortably fit, and in which their wishes will be better assured, while adding additional continuity between the acute and postacute settings.

Although the DNR order is the most common type of "withholding" order, orders to withhold or withdraw other medical procedures are arising with much greater frequency than formerly. As a result of this and the Joint Commission's monitoring of withholding of medical life-prolonging procedures, questions about medical appropriateness, legal and ethical considerations, public policy, and even cost are being taken more seriously.

There is a range of misperceptions about what "DNR" or "No Code" means. Furthermore, clinicians, lawyers, and administrators have realized that the primacy given to DNR orders is often misplaced. Lack of a broad-based policy has resulted in confusion about whether a DNR order encompasses life-prolonging medical procedures such as vasopressors, palliative interventions, and mechanical ventilation as well as the whens, hows, and under what circumstances what should be done. This confusion is exacerbated by the fact that we have granted withholding cardiac and/or pulmonary resuscitation a special status and have even assigned it special names ("No Code," "DNR"). Using "withholding cardiac and/or pulmonary resuscitation" as one instance in a wider range of "withholding issues" instead of "DNR" is not only clearer and more accurate but guards against and prevents unnecessary uncertainty and confusion.

The question whether to withhold or withdraw life-prolonging medical procedures is often seen mainly as a legal rather than a medical issue. Although there are obvious legal and ethical components, the question is fundamentally medical in nature. Withholding or withdrawing treatment in a case where the prognosis or diagnosis is unclear makes little sense. A variety of medical factors, including the prognosis, the likely efficacy of the proposed intervention, and the appropriateness of alternatives, must be integrated into the decision-making process.

Following is an integrated policy on the withholding or withdrawing of life-prolonging medical procedures. A policy of this type must be tailored to the particular institution that adopts it.

POLICY ON WITHHOLDING/WITHDRAWING LIFE-PROLONGING PROCEDURES

Purpose

The purpose of this policy is to provide general guidance for the hospital and medical staff for withholding or withdrawing life-prolonging medical procedures. Adults with the capacity to make medical decisions have the right to actively participate in decision making. This right of self-determination includes treatment decisions as well as decisions to withhold or withdraw life-prolonging procedures.

The facility recognizes both the importance of maintaining patient self-determination as well as the importance of offering realistic and viable medical options. The physician should identify several factors when considering writing an order to withhold or withdraw life-prolonging medical procedures including potential benefit, prognosis, morbidity, and the patient's expressed wishes regarding medical intervention and end-of-life decisions. The attending physician should participate in the decision-making process by making specific recommendations and defining reasonable alternatives based on viable medical options for the patient and/or acceptable surrogate.

These guidelines are intended to assist the physician, support the patient's self-determination, and reduce conflict; they neither exclude nor replace the exercise of the physician's clinical judgment, particularly in situations that arise unexpectedly and are potentially reversible. Such situations should be discussed with the patient in advance.

Withholding Cardiac or Pulmonary Resuscitation (No Code)

1. A "No Code" order refers specifically to withholding cardiac or pulmonary resuscitation. All other modalities for symptom control, such as those intended to reduce pain, prevent seizures, and provide comfort, should be implemented as needed.

2. A No Code order may be considered when (a) there is a terminal condition with no reasonable hope for recovery; (b) the patient is in the late stages of an ongoing deteriorative disease; or (c) the patient has specifically expressed a wish, either directly or through an advance directive or an acceptable surrogate, not to be resuscitated.

3. Discussion of a No Code order is preferably initiated by the attending physician (or his or her designate) or the patient. However, a surrogate decision maker or another clinician may initiate the discussion as well.

4. After the No Code order has been written and properly documented in the medical record, resuscitative measures will not be initiated in the event of cardiac or pulmonary arrest.

5. The attending physician (or designate) is responsible for (a) discussing the No Code order with the patient and, when appropriate, the family or an acceptable nonfamilial surrogate; (b) documenting ongoing discussions and decisions in the medical record; and (c) periodically assessing the No Code order.

6. A No Code order is not an endpoint but often sets the stage for a wide range of other decisions, including those involving the withholding or withdrawing of other life-prolonging medical procedures.

Withholding or Withdrawing Other Life-Prolonging Medical Procedures

1. Life-prolonging medical procedures include medication administration and artificially or technologically supplied respiration, nutrition, and hydration when such procedures serve only to prolong the dying process.

2. An order to withhold or withdraw life-prolonging medical procedures may be considered when (a) there is a terminal condition with no reasonable hope for recovery; (b) the patient is in the late stages of an ongoing deteriorative or degenerative disease; or (c) the patient has expressed a wish, either directly or through an ad-

vance directive or an acceptable surrogate, not to undergo such procedures.

3. Discussions of such an order should be initiated by the attending physician (or his or her designate), the patient, the family, or an acceptable nonfamilial surrogate.

4. Appropriate referrals should be made to confirm medical status and prognosis before a withhold/withdraw order is written by the attending physician.

5. The patient's physician is responsible for (a) discussing the withhold/withdraw order with the patient and, when appropriate, the family or an acceptable nonfamilial surrogate; (b) documenting ongoing discussions and decisions in the medical record; and (c) ongoing assessment of the withhold/withdraw order.

6. All other treatment modalities, such as those intended to reduce pain, prevent seizures, and provide comfort, should be implemented as needed.

Medically Futile Condition

1. If the attending physician determines that the patient's condition is terminal, and there is no hope of recovery, it follows that any attempted resuscitation or life support would be futile even if provided and would therefore be fundamentally inappropriate.

2. Ongoing discussion of the patient's condition is important as part of the anticipatory grief process if further intervention is determined to be medically inappropriate.

3. The patient's chart shall contain documentation of the basis for the determination of medical futility, the physician's written orders to withhold or withdraw resuscitation or life support, and documentation of attempts to notify family members.

Procedures: Medical Assessment and Documentation

Medical Assessment

1. A No Code or Withhold/Withdraw order should include a comprehensive assessment by the physician

primarily responsible for the patient's care and be documented in the medical record. Reasonable efforts should be made to confirm medical status with appropriate referrals.

2. As in any other clinical decision, a No Code or Withhold/Withdraw order should be re-evaluated periodically based on the medical status and specific circumstances of the patient.

Documentation

1. The No Code or Withhold/Withdraw order must be written and approved by the attending physician (or his or her designate) on the physician's order sheet and in the progress notes. This order must be signed and dated.

2. Ongoing discussions with the patient, the family, or an acceptable nonfamilial surrogate should be documented in the progress notes (included should be the date, time, and significant content of such discussions). Any specific declarations made by the patient directly or by the patient to the family or an acceptable nonfamilial surrogate should be documented in the medical record. Such information can help ensure the self-determination of the patient is respected and resolve potential conflict.

3. There are special circumstances when a telephone order for No Code may be appropriate. A telephone order for No Code must be documented, dated, and signed by two clinicians.

4. There are circumstances in which a No Code or Withhold/Withdraw order may be temporarily suspended during a specific invasive procedure (e.g., palliative surgery or a diagnostic procedure). Any proposed changes (including a temporary suspension) in a No Code or Withhold/Withdraw order should be discussed with the patient, the family, or an acceptable nonfamilial surrogate and documented in the medical record.

5. The patient or an authorized surrogate acting in the patient's stead may request a change in a No Code or Withhold/Withdraw order at any time.

Conflict Resolution

The patient's wishes should be honored provided that these wishes are consistent with the ethical integrity of the medical profession and the patient understands and appreciates the significance of his or her wishes.

However, there may be circumstances when the patient's wishes are unknown or unclear or there is unresolved conflict among surrogate decision makers. In such circumstances, the following mechanisms are suggested to resolve any conflict:

1. Contact the patient representative department to initiate a conflict resolution process.
2. Family or pastoral care conferences may be requested to assist in resolving the conflict.
3. Disagreement among physicians and other caregivers should be resolved prior to any discussions with the patient, the family, or an acceptable nonfamilial surrogate. Other medical professionals, medical staff committee members, department heads, and hospital administrators may be consulted to help resolve the conflict.
4. If the conflict remains unresolved, then the hospital ethics committee may be consulted. The ethics committee may consult with the legal counsel if appropriate.
5. The patient's wishes documented during former hospitalizations or treatment at other health care settings can serve as a helpful guide for conflict resolution and future decision making.

Related Provisions

1. When the patient is unable to make health care decisions and his or her wishes regarding specific decisions are unknown, then an acceptable surrogate may act in his or her behalf. In making any health care decision for the patient, the surrogate shall consider the recommendation of the attending physician, any evidence as to what the patient would have decided if the patient had decisional capacity, and what decision would be in the best interest of the patient.
2. Following is the order of priority for surrogate health care decision makers: (1) a person with a valid medical durable power of attorney, (2) a legal guardian with au-

thority for making medical decisions, (3) a validly des-ignated health care surrogate, (4) the patient's spouse, (5) adult children of age, (6) either parent, or (7) adult brothers or sisters. Those who can provide a reasonable indication of the patient's views can offer helpful direction for decision-making purposes.

3. If, for reasons of conscience, any caregiver cannot comply with a Withhold/Withdraw order or with the patient's specific wishes, the caregiver must notify the appropriate department head or medical staff director of the refusal or inability to comply so that appropriate measures can be taken.

4 .Advance directives, such as a living will, a medical durable power of attorney, or a patient-drafted directive, may be helpful guides for decision making and are usually considered to indicate patient intent. They can be critical in preventing or resolving conflict.

CASE STUDIES

Case 1

Ms. D., a nurse and ethics committee member, has read extensively in the medical and nursing ethics literature and is aware that many people believe there is no ethical difference between withholding and withdrawing life-prolonging medical procedures. Yet she also knows by experience that when life-prolonging procedures are going to be withdrawn, special safeguards are instituted. Documentation becomes more detailed, the ethics committee is always consulted, and each step in the process is subjected to extra scrutiny.

- Doesn't the extra care taken show that there *is* a difference between withholding life-prolonging treatment and withdrawing treatment that has already been put into place?
- If there is a difference, what implications would it have for patient care?
- What implications would it have for policy development?
- What implications does this have for caring for patients?

Case 2

An integrated delivery system offers a wide range of postacute services. The agency has been the target of several malpractice suits and has learned the importance of developing guiding policies. In an effort to avert problems, it has implemented very restrictive policies, and as a condition of admission into its program patients must agree to live within the boundaries of these policies. Many standard patient rights are therefore not honored.

- Do policies that infringe on a patient's rights have validity?
- If a patient wanted to become a client of the agency's but did not want to give up his or her rights, what options would the patient have?

Case 3

A patient has indicated he does not want to be resuscitated should he suffer cardiac or pulmonary arrest. One of the nurses has developed a close relationship with the patient and has talked with him about his wishes regarding DNR. She knows that the patient's physician has a reputation for overriding or ignoring the wishes of patients not to be resuscitated when they can no longer express themselves. The physician has strong religious convictions and believes it is always better to "err on the side of life."

- Should the nurse inform the patient or family members about the physician's reputation?
- If she does nothing, will she be guilty of legal or ethical negligence?
- How should the physician be dealt with?
- What role could the ethics committee play in helping to ensure the patient's autonomy?

Case 4

Mr. W. is admitted to a hospital emergency department because of a severe sore throat. The resident who takes the history overlooks some important information and fails to realize the seriousness of the symptoms. Appropriate tests are not performed and Mr. W.'s condition deteriorates dramatically.

Because of the incompetence of the resident and the unfortunate consequences of the misdiagnosis, Mr. W.'s family transfers him to another facility. His condition is evaluated and his family is told that he may be in a persistent vegetative state. Because this diagnosis has not been confirmed and Mr. W. may be experiencing pain, analgesics are prescribed and administered through a syringe.

Several days pass and Mr. W.'s condition does not seem to change. The family is beginning to come to grips with the fact that he may never regain consciousness. One of the sons, more outspoken than the other children, asserts that Mr. W.'s time to die has come and requests that a lethal dose of some drug be administered. The staff refuse to consider this request seriously because it is perceived to be contrary to the ethics of the profession and illegal as well. The son who asked for the lethal dose becomes very sullen and even shows hostility toward the nurses when they enter Mr. W.'s room to check on him and give him the analgesic. Family members have even attempted to encourage the nurse to leave the syringe with its remaining contents behind. The family members are not mean-spirited but want to end Mr. W.'s life as he would have wanted. The nurses are concerned that the son might try to take events into his own hands and do something to end Mr. W.'s life.

- What should the nurses do in this situation?
- What role might the ethics committee be able to play?
- What are the main ethical issues at stake? The main legal issues?
- What is the physician's responsibility?

Case 5

A surgeon who is consistently up to date on new technologies has been using a laser procedure that is less invasive, less expensive, and safer than conventional surgical procedures. She wants to use it to treat a patient who is a member of a managed care organization which does not pay for the new procedure. The physician attempts to get special permission but the managed care organization refuses her request. The surgeon performs the novel procedure but bills for a covered procedure. She wants to do the right thing but she also wants to get paid. She believes she should not provide inferior care solely because the insurer is behind the times.

- What is the central ethical issue?
- What should an administrator do if he or she discovers the fraud? Would it make a difference if the administrator believes the new procedure is in fact preferable?
- Should the surgeon put the patient at risk because of an outdated payment policy?

8

Conducting an Ethics Audit

REVIEWING POLICIES AND ENSURING CONSISTENCY

In order to create or upgrade an ethics program in a facility or an agency, it is important to assess organizational strengths and weaknesses. This includes investigating the organization's history, identifying past cases or situations that could serve as a basis for education, and uncovering any impediments to establishing or refining such a program. It is also important to identify past successes and to institute policies that will create an appropriate environment for addressing ethical concerns.

One of the first steps is to perform an "ethics audit." One of the goals of such an audit is to determine whether policies are consistent across departments. It is not uncommon for hospital departments to have contradictory ways of dealing with the same issues. For example, a DNR order might be honored in most departments but might be ignored or temporarily suspended without patient permission during palliative surgery. When people use a policy in an inconsistent fashion, it invalidates the policy and reduces its effectiveness. A policy is intended to provide consistency and direction, and any deviation from the policy must be explained and documented.

Knowing and acting in accordance with facility policies is an important part of medical and nursing practice. "Doing the right thing," if inconsistent with a stated policy, increases the facility's liability exposure and creates confusion. Inconsistency spawns invalidation of a policy, be the policy good or bad. For example, policies that ensure the wishes and rights of patients need to be honored at all stages of patient care, not just in critical situations or at the end of life. Policies should be consistent across facility lines to better assure continuity of patients' wishes across the continuum.

137

When refining or upgrading policies, it is extremely important to purge them of ambiguous or archaic language. Words like "heroic," for example, have little meaning today. Replacing "heroic" or "heroic measures" with language like the American Medical Association Council on Ethical and Judicial Affairs uses (e.g., "life-prolonging medical treatment or procedures when such treatment or procedures prolong the dying process") is appropriate. It is not uncommon to see policies that say that in the absence of a DNR order, the care providers should "err towards life." This is a strange notion. I suggest not that we should "err" towards death, but that we should not err at all. Using erring as a clinical guideline is extremely suspect. If it is clearly medically inappropriate to resuscitate a patient, then having such a provision in place creates nothing but uncertainty and potential legal exposure.

Having transfer policies to ensure continuity of consent and of care is important, as is having a conflict resolution policy. An ethics audit should include an evaluation of these policies as well as policies regarding end-of-life decision making.

EVALUATING CONFLICT RESOLUTION TECHNIQUES

There are many different ways to address conflict. One important rule is to avoid jumping to the last step first—to go to court and look for a legal solution. The first attempt at conflict resolution should be between the patient (or surrogate) and the caregiver. Identifying impediments to resolving issues and controversies, clearing up misconceptions, and identifying other blockages to decision making are often fruitful tactics. If they are insufficient, there are other intrainstitutional resources to call upon to stimulate the resolution process.

In-house conflict resolution mechanisms are preferable to external mechanisms. At times, however, bringing in an outsider may be in order. I have frequently given lectures to reluctant medical and nursing staff who have misconceptions about or discomfort with conflict resolution. These lectures have been used to get the ball rolling on the right path or at least in the right direction. The usual internal tools for resolving conflict are (interdisciplinary) patient care conferences, pastoral care conferences, and family conferences with the social work department.

Evaluating an existing formal mechanism or procedure for resolving conflict or creating one is another step in an ethics audit. A conflict resolution policy should define how conflict should be addressed, by whom, and under what circumstances. Below are some guidelines that should be kept in mind when devising a conflict resolution policy.

CONFLICT RESOLUTION GUIDELINES

The following guidelines should be used in case of conflict, whether it involves caregivers, family members, the patient, or the patient's surrogate:

1. *Conflict is ideally resolved through opportunities for informal but enhanced communication between the parties.*
2. *Involvement of a third party, such as a supervisor, an administrator, or a risk manager, can increase the likelihood of a resolution.*
3. *If a conflict arises between the patient (or surrogate) and representatives of the facility, the following should be considered:*
   — A pastoral care conference might be initiated. Pastoral care staff can be most helpful in addressing problems of denial, unresolved grief, religious perceptions and misperceptions, and impediments to decision making.
   — Involving a social worker in family conferences can be beneficial. Often decision making is impeded by concern or frustration on the part of family members, who may be worried that they will not be able to meet the patient's needs at home.
   Both social workers and pastoral care staff can be of assistance in the conflict resolution process. Which to use first depends on the given circumstances and the availability of personnel. Both can enlist other individuals in the agency or facility to assist in decision making as well as offer the family the option of convening the ethics committee. It is not uncommon for social workers and pastoral care staff to be on the ethics committee and to be able to identify the resources needed for a timely resolution of conflict.

4. *Ethics rounds and consultations can assist in bedside problem solving.* The ethics committee should be a forum for identifying problems and resolving current or precluding future conflict. It can also help create educational opportunities for staff and surrogate decision makers and interpret policies and procedures for anyone who is unclear about these.

5. *Consulting the legal counsel is sometimes an important step in the conflict resolution process.* The legal counsel can identify or clarify policy provisions, highlight ambiguities and inconsistencies, and suggest future directions. Also, if reasonable attempts to address a conflict using internal processes fail, the legal counsel can evaluate whether the probate system or another external mechanism might be appropriate. Note that consulting the legal counsel, except for clarification of a policy issue, is generally not one of the early steps in the conflict resolution process.

Devising or modifying policies is meaningless if the ethics program lacks an educational component. Committee members, staff, and patients and family members all need to be informed about the policies that apply in given circumstances.

In addition, how policies and procedures are created is critical to their effectiveness and whether staff assume ownership of them. Staff must understand why the policies exist and what the process is for deciding which issues need to be addressed through the creation of policies. They also need to learn to appreciate the complexity and diversity of perspectives and distinctive approaches to dealing with the issues of self-determination and decisional competence, and accept their responsibility for creating a supportive environment in which patients and surrogates can make informed decisions. In addition, care providers need to educate each other on ethical issues and let each other know that such issues are of grave importance to them.

Ethics consultants can help resolve conflict by providing clarification on specific questions or dilemmas and identifying pertinent resources or materials. They can also assist in policy development, anticipate problems that might arise on a regular basis, and provide educational opportunities within the development process.

CASE STUDIES

Case 1

Mrs. T. now lacks decisional capacity and has never identified a health care agent. Family members have been repeatedly informed that death is near and have prepared for the inevitable. Each time, however, Mrs. T. rallies and regains strength. The family members have become frustrated because she will not die "on time." They wish the best for her but her dying process has become costly both in terms of time and money and also is emotionally draining for them. Mrs. T. has been evaluated as having an intermittent swallowing disorder and cannot always eat. The family members ask the physician to write an order to stop feeding her.

- What responsibility does the physician have?
- What responsibility does the administrative director have?
- Should the family members' inconvenience be a criterion in the medical management of this case?
- What role might a surrogate play in this situation?
- Is the guardianship a consideration? Why or why not?

Case 2

Mr. K. is terminally ill. He has no remaining family and has not chosen a surrogate decision maker. He is an alcoholic and has lived in the same apartment for 15 years. The person closest to him is his landlord, who has seen him through his drinking binges, visits him regularly, and has been a vital source of help.

- Does the landlord have any legal standing as a surrogate decision maker?
- Can the landlord legitimately assist in decision making? Why or why not?
- What is the goal of surrogate decision making?
- Would assigning a guardian be an appropriate means of identifying the patient's wishes?

9

Clinical Ethics Rounds

For a facility unwilling, or for some reason, unable to create an ethics committee, clinical ethics rounds may serve as a helpful vehicle to address ethical issues. It is also an excellent teaching resource and a valuable addition to an ethics committee if one exists. Ethics rounds constitute a more natural forum for open discussion than an ethics committee, which is more public in nature. Through active and ongoing participation in ethics rounds, clinicians can become better educated and gain mastery in dealing with problems and issues that otherwise would create great discomfort.

Unit- or agency-based ethics rounds have many advantages over an ethics committee as a means of dealing with controversy in a timely fashion. Departmental ethics rounds should be offered at least monthly, with interim ad hoc meetings as required. Attendance is not obligatory, and care providers need not attend every meeting to keep up with issues and solutions, for the content of such rounds is informally transmitted quickly and easily.

Whereas an ethics committee, or any hospital committee for that matter, has the luxury of being able to carefully sort through alternatives, ethics rounds are a boon to the clinician who must make a decision immediately. Having other individuals involved in thinking about a difficult issue can be very helpful. The clinician can accept the assistance of peers without losing face and without having to make his or her confusion or indecisiveness known to a large number of people. Furthermore, all of those on the rounds learn the insights and critical skills that each caregiver is able to bring to a decision-making process.

Ethics rounds may be integrated into regular clinical rounds or they may occur as a separate educational tool. In the latter case, rounds often last approximately one to one and a half hours and occur at least twice a month, with ad hoc meetings as requested. High-tech settings and critical care services often require more frequent meetings.

Ethics rounds can consist of a roundtable discussion in an informal setting where medical and nursing staff can float in and out as their schedules permit or they can be a component of patient care or even case management rounds. Specific presentations may be scheduled to clarify a certain issue endemic to the type of the decision being contemplated or to explicate certain facets of decision making. There is almost always informal discussion after each session, and, when indicated, chart notations are made concerning suggestions or modifications in care plans resulting from the session.

THE BENEFITS OF ETHICS ROUNDS

As already noted, an ethics committee is extremely important for the effectiveness of ethics rounds, for a policy in place can preclude many of the recurrent problems that arise. However, although the ethics committee can develop a policy on the withholding or withdrawing of life-prolonging medical procedures, what about that attending who never can make a final decision about the prognosis of a patient and thus puts the family through a long period of misery and confusion? The problems that arise in this kind of situation can be minimized if other caregivers are provided the chance to discuss them and try to arrive at reasonable solutions, which is exactly what ethics rounds are intended to do—provide that chance.

Take, for example, a situation in which a patient has indicated that he does not want to be resuscitated should he go into cardiac arrest. He tells his physician that his wife and all surviving relatives will not agree with him and he seeks assurance that the physician will honor his wish. When he deteriorates and becomes incompetent, the physician will be tempted to act in accordance with what the family members want, motivated to some extent by the knowledge that the survivors are the ones in a position to sue. What should the physician do? What should the nurse do?

If the ethics committee has developed and adopted a clear policy that addresses this and related issues, the caregivers will have better guidance and better insulation. The policy might indicate that the stated wishes of a patient will not be allowed to be thwarted, undermined, or compromised by any third parties, including family members. It might also define what steps should be taken to resolve a conflict of this type. Such a policy would help the physician honor the patient's wish and feel secure in so doing.

Of course, ethics rounds might also help. Other caregivers might suggest to the physician that he take the following steps: (1) chart the disparity between what the competent patient wants and what the family members want; (2) request a family conference and chart the results (via the department of social work); and (3) request that pastoral care be called in and chart their involvement. In taking these steps, the physician will increase his protection if he chooses (as he should) to honor the wishes of the patient. If he wants to do this but is still uneasy, he could ask for a consultation to determine whether the patient is competent to make a medical decision. Regardless of whether guidance comes from an ethics committee or ethics rounds, it will be a help in dealing with ongoing problems and avoiding mistakes.

Again, suppose an attending physician is reluctant to perform a given task (such as the writing of a DNR order). What would likely happen if a colleague brought this problem to the attention of the ethics committee? Her ability to work with the attending could well become compromised and the seeds of future interprofessional conflict might be planted. Yet the attending's continued reluctance is causing problems for the patient's family and the hospital staff. Now suppose the ethics committee has developed good policies on consent, DNR orders, and withholding or withdrawing other life-prolonging medical procedures. Further suppose that the issue of the attending's reluctance is raised for discussion during ethics rounds. The administrator or medical director would then be able to intervene without interloping, because all he or she would be doing is bringing the already established hospital policy to the attention of the physician and giving fair warning that failure to act in accordance with the policy could create potential problems, including a charge of malpractice.

Departmental ethics rounds offer a means for discussing and addressing recurring issues fruitfully. They should not serve as a mechanism for pursuing business as usual or for evading troublesome problems and issues. In fact, ethics rounds tend to force issues to the fore. They provide an opportunity to talk formally about problems that are causing mere grumbling and can make explicit what has been to date only implicit.

CLINICAL ETHICS ROUNDS AND THE ETHICS COMMITTEE

The relationship between ethics rounds and the ethics committee is important to understand. Obviously, the better equipped the rounds members are to address controversies and dilemmas and the better they know the institution's or agency's policies, the more effective they will be in ensuring the policies are adopted and followed. The rounds can help the ethics committee identify the need for policy development by bringing recurrent problems to its attention. Since the rounds are usually open only to care team members, some mechanism for getting information to the other services may be needed. However, they need not be limited to clinicians.

One good strategy is to include a representative from legal services on the rounds so as to get legal perspective. In addition, having an in-house lawyer and a risk manager present will be of value when it comes to developing institutional policies, since they will better understand clinical issues and appreciate the dynamics of providing medical services. By bringing together clinicians and lawyers in a context where they can educate each other and learn to work together, ethics rounds can increase the likelihood that institutional policies and problem solving will be more effective and more practical.

Ethics rounds also offer a forum for clarifying and addressing guideline issues. If the facility has adopted guidelines but certain situations do not seem to be covered by the guidelines, the hospital attorney, after learning about the problem from attending the rounds, can bring it to the attention of the appropriate person and make suggestions for modifications.

ETHICS ROUNDS AND DISCOVERABILITY

It is currently an open question whether ethics committee discussions must be recorded and whether the minutes are discoverable or covered by the umbrella of peer review. In many cases, I think that some of the proceedings of an ethics committee may indeed be discoverable, depending on what information is requested and why. Others have argued that if the ethics committee proceedings are part of the quality assurance process, then they are not discoverable, particularly when there is a peer review component. Clinical discussions during ethics rounds, however, need not be documented and minutes are not taken. Minutes are never taken for clinical discussions or rounds, so this is no deviance from accepted policy, nor could it be perceived as an attempt to hide information.

ETHICS ROUNDS AND ADJUDICATING CONFLICT

There is another critical function that ethics rounds can perform—assisting in the development of policies in areas where distinctive or novel issues arise in a given setting or unit. For example, in many hospitals a high percentage of ICU beds are filled with nursing home residents, some of whom are in persistent vegetative states. As a consequence, patients who could benefit from treatment in an ICU are prevented from getting a bed.

Suppose a hospital ethics committee wishes to address this issue, which was brought to its attention by participants in the ICU ethics rounds. Since the ethics rounds participants are used to working together to define and resolve problems, they would be exceptionally well qualified to play a major role in developing a policy regarding the use of ICU beds for patients with long-term acute care needs.

Other issues arise from the "trampoline effect"—the repeated transfer of patients from the hospital to the nursing home and back again. For example, how do caregivers ensure that a patient's wishes will be honored when he or she is transferred from one facility to another? The patient's chart does not accompany the patient, and a mere discharge summary that says the patient is a DNR might not be adequate. This continuity of care issue is an example of the issues that ethics rounds can help to address.

Ethics rounds offer an informal environment for identifying or talking about ethical issues. They can enhance the effectiveness of a given service and the ethics committee as well. Having an ethics committee is not a prerequisite for holding ethics rounds, but such a committee, unlike ethics rounds, can develop policies that will help caregivers resolve recurrent avoidable problems.

CASE STUDIES

Case 1

A physician orders home physical therapy for an adolescent with long bone fractures. The physical therapist knows that providing this modality to the patient will stimulate bone growth significantly—to such an extent, in fact, that the one leg will be longer than the other. The physician does not realize the danger. The physical therapist, who has been only recently certified, is uncomfortable challenging the prescription of a senior member of the medical staff. She provides the therapy but never turns the machine on. She also tears up the bill.

- Do her actions solve the problem? Why or why not?
- What are the ethical issues in this case?
- How can such issues best be addressed?

Case 2

Mr. L. has indicated that he does not want to be resuscitated. Several years ago a close friend of his who had stopped breathing for 30 minutes was resuscitated by emergency medical technicians. Since then he has been in a persistent vegetative state. Mr. L. heard that the longest recorded case of someone in a persistent vegetative state was 37 years and 111 days and he does not want to end up the same way. As a safeguard, he has drafted an advance directive saying he does not want to be intubated or to have chest compressions or pressors and the like under any circumstance. He has an acute apneac episode believed to be associated with a mucous plug.

- What should the nurse do?
- What role, if any, might the ethics committee play?
- What role might a patient care, pastoral care, or family conference play?

- How can Mr. L.'s caregivers address his concerns and give him the confidence to let them deal with acutely reversible events?
- What role could ethics rounds play?
- What implications does this have for avoiding "doing everything" and "doing nothing " discourse?

10

The Facility-Based Ethics Committee

There is increased pressure to create formal mechanisms for conflict resolution and policy development in health care facilities. Ethics committees can be helpful in dealing with ethical issues. They can also be used to mend the seams of the delivery system to better ensure continuity of care as well as continuity of patients' wishes. However, questions as to their value, role, and scope need to be answered fully. Also, existing committees can become stagnant and purposeless and need revitalization.

Establishing an ethics committee—an institutional forum for addressing a wide range of ethical issues—is not always an easy task. Like many innovative mechanisms for addressing controversy, an ethics committee may be feared as potentially too influential, and its role may be reduced from problem solving to identification of and education about ethical issues. Many committees were actually set up primarily for educational purposes.

HISTORY OF ETHICS COMMITTEES

Historically, ethics committees were created, not to solve systemic institutional problems, but to solve a specific problem in an acute care setting. Over time, however, fora for addressing a wide range of medical and administrative issues emerged. Few have arisen in long-term care facilities, where there is less support and less medical guidance than exists in a hospital and where end-of-life issues are often more subtle.

The first legal use of an ethics committee to resolve an end-of-life issue occurred in *Quinlan*. The court made use of a medical prognosis committee composed of physicians who speculated as to the prognosis based on their clinical findings. This medical prognosis committee was widely misinterpreted to be an ethics committee—a committee that could appropriately address a wide range of difficult legal and ethical questions.

The use in *Quinlan* of a medical prognosis committee, despite or perhaps because of the misunderstanding of its nature, fueled the desire of many practitioners to institute an ethics forum. On the other hand, many physicians, fearing that their clinical decisions might be questioned, did not want such a forum. Other vehicles for physician oversight, such as quality assurance and risk management committees, were also viewed negatively by many in the medical community. As a result, the ethics committees that were created were reluctant to encroach on the turf of clinicians and thus remained relatively ineffective.

Most of the ethics committees that have been successful have built upon their work in dealing with DNR issues and have avoided an advisory role. Advisory committees tend to be perceived by physicians as unwelcomed intruders and as a source of additional stress in an already nerve-racking situation.

New pressures have created a need to re-evaluate the scope and mission of ethics committees. Although resolving clinical and administrative conflict became a fruitful role for many committees, current conflicts have expanded far beyond the intrainstitutional bickering of the past. Health care reform and the drive toward managed care have admitted patients, courts, insurers, and even politicians into the wrestling ring. Systemic issues, including questions regarding what services can be provided to whom and when, have grown in importance. It is these issues that present an opportunity for ethics committees to expand their role, not only in hospitals, where discussion of these issues is relatively mature, but also in long-term care facilities and home health agencies, which are relatively inexperienced in dealing with the constraints imposed by managed care.

ETHICS COMMITTEES AND EDUCATION

Ethics committees have often been labelled as "advisory," which means their function is to encourage the physicians through education to "do the right thing." I believe there was an assumption that rational solutions to ethical dilemmas would somehow float to the top and magically display them-selves so clearly that physicians could not help but do what was right. Another assumption was that ethics committees, by deliberating on ethical issues, would become so adept at solving problems that they could deal with the very complex problems beginning to arise in high-technology medicine.

To play their proper role, ethics committee members must

- gain some sense of what ethics is all about
- understand the role, scope, and charge of the committee
- identify the strengths and weaknesses of the committee
- master problem identification, problem solving, and conflict resolution techniques
- know how to test and refine provisional decisions or recommendations
- recognize that there will not necessarily be clearly defined right and wrong answers but that the problem-solving process itself can be helpful and illuminating
- learn how to clarify or flesh out important components of a problem and explore an array of solutions to identify the most appropriate one
- recognize that getting together to talk about a problem and merely feeling better as a result is not a sufficient response to the problem
- understand the ethical and legal issues that often arise in case discussion and policy development

ETHICS COMMITTEES AND ADVOCACY

The traditional role ethics committees have played in education and policy development is often complemented by their expanding role as advocates for health care providers when external constraints compromise the delivery of care or services to patients. Patient advocacy, of course, has become a byword of the health care reform movement. Both the American Medical Association and the American Hospital Association, for example, place a greater emphasis on advocacy than in the past. The role of advocate for patients and providers is somewhat different than the role assumed by prototypical ethics committees.

LONG-TERM CARE AND HOME HEALTH ETHICS COMMITTEES

Although many highly trained clinical specialists spend an inordinate amount of time getting administrative approval to treat from third-party payers, long-term and home care providers, who have less credibility than physicians, often find the approval process almost unfathomable. The role of oversight by government agencies exacerbates the challenge and may create regulatory disincentives that do not exist in the hospital. For example, although most hospitals are required to provide staffing "appropriate to the needs of the patient," long-term care regulations will usually specify the number of hours each day and even the times during the day that various levels of care must be provided. Procedures and services that are discretionary in a hospital, such as evening snacks for patients, are required in a long-term care facility. Thus, long-term care facilities lack the flexibility to plan effective and efficient health care for their residents in a managed care atmosphere.

In addition, long-term care facilities are perceived as "warehouses" for the elderly, and the health professionals who work in them are often viewed as more concerned about making money than about providing care. The reality that government reimbursement is limited but government service demands are vast is hardly ever mentioned in the public debate on health care. Thus having a forum, such as an ethics committee, to increase their credibility is becoming a necessity for many long-term care providers. They need opportunities for input and negotiation to combat the pressure from managed care organizations to compromise care.

For example, managed care organizations may mandate that physicians in long-term care be board-certified geriatricians. This would exclude many physicians currently working in long-term care facilities and may put them out of business. The facilities, on the other hand, may be unable to attract and pay for board-certified specialists to oversee the care provided to their residents and may be forced to close.

It is difficult to obtain accurate and up-to-date information on ethics committees in long-term and home care delivery environments, but it is clear that, unlike the crisis management model found in many hospitals, they have a more expansive role as a forum for developing policies that affect the daily lives of residents and patients. At the same time, although facilities and agencies are encouraged to address ethical issues by the Omnibus Budget Reconciliation Act of 1991, there may be sufficient financial disincentives to impede or even undermine the process. For example, reimbursement for both home care and long-term care is currently based primarily on the costs incurred by the provider. In order to increase reimbursement, the provider must provide more care. Thus it is not in the provider's best interest to cease providing care by not resuscitating a patient. Likewise, the mandate to implement a process of advance directives for residents and clients is unfunded. The costs in terms of time, effort, forms, and recordkeeping are not reimbursed by the government and therefore detract from an often slim bottom line. There must be positive incentives for ethics issues to be fully and properly explored in long-term and home care settings. Perhaps the recognition that increasingly verdicts are being rendered against providers for the failiure to honor advance directives will help correct this. A Genessee County, Michigan jury returned a $6.6 million verdict against a Flint, Michigan hospital that kept Brenda Young on life support against her family's wishes.[1]

An ethics committee can be especially helpful in addressing medical futility issues. Family members often demand that providers do something that is medically inappropriate. Their requests usually stem from misunderstandings caused by earlier transactions (perhaps an exhausted staff physician carelessly asked, "If his heart stops, do you want us to start it?"). Essential questions, such as those regarding quality of life, informed consent, and the patient's wishes, are often forgotten in the heat of the emergency. When faced with the reality of death, the family members only remember that the caregiver was going to restart the heart. If in ethics committee meetings staff have been sensitized to the need to engage in real discussions with patients and family members as well as interact among themselves to reach a consensus regarding consent, the likelihood of adverse legal consequences and bad public relations can be minimized.

ETHICS COMMITTEES AND THE COMMUNITY

I believe that a properly utilized ethics committee will be seen by care providers as an asset, not just another watchdog. When a facility is faced with a difficult decision that carries the potential for regulatory penalties or even a civil or criminal lawsuit, it is important to have community support on its side. Many complaints occur when acute care staff, who often do not understand the nature of chronically debilitating illnesses, are presented with a patient in a condition that they assume must have been caused by negligence in the long-term care setting. Having a representative from the local hospital emergency room on the facility's ethics committee can help foster open discussion of the many clinical differences that characterize the two settings and eliminate or reduce the misunderstandings that inevitably occur.

Likewise, when a facility is faced with adverse action in a hostile regulatory environment, having the community leadership on its side is often crucial for survival. Hostile regulators fail to provide even the slightest hint of how to provide superior care while living within regulatory constraints. Once a violation of regulations has been cited, the regulators refuse to even communicate with the facility or to revisit it to carry out their mandated overwatch functions until the legal process is completed, often months later. The only way to avert this incomprehensible block is to ask local, regional, or state lawmakers to intercede. If they or their staffs have been involved with the facility through the ethics committee process, they will provide their help willingly and promptly. What more incentive can a long-term care facility want than help when it is needed?

Whatever issues are being considered by an ethics committee may also eventually be considered in the wider community. For example, even though confidentiality is of paramount importance, it must be considered in light of the need of care providers to share information to create a seamless delivery system. While protection of patient information is critical, the sharing of information actually enhances patient care by transmitting critical patient data from one health care setting to another. The high ideals of the community can be influential and may help shape legislation and even national policy, but the day-to-day issues that make life better for residents and staff should be the main focus of committee discussions. Community concerns about resource allocation, access to care, and cost must be brought to the committee by community representatives, and the committee's (and facility's) responses should be publicized in return.

Although managed care organizations and long-term care facilities may sometimes act like adversaries, it still might make sense to have a managed care representative on an ethics committee in order to minimize miscommunication and create commonality of purpose. Working together allows facility and nonfacility committee members to learn how to frame problems and issues so as to engender community understanding and acceptance. If there is a foundation of community support, there is a greater likelihood of shared initiatives, shared responsibility, and shared accountability. Perhaps this could turn back the movement toward a situation where each institution has its own policies and those policies are incongruent with the policies of other institutions, which of course creates tremendous confusion for patients and caregivers. Replacing the morass of conflicting policies with sensible policies that are shared across health care boundaries and creating a truly seamless health care delivery system should be the goal of every ethics committee.

Marketing has not usually been seen as a natural offshoot of an ethics program. This blindness has led to many missed opportunities. Patients do not always know which is the "best place" for them to go. An important criterion in their decision where to go is that they feel comfortable with the policies of the facility and believe that the staff will work with them, listen to them, and respond to their fears and anxiety. In short, they are looking for a place they can trust. Knowing that a facility has an ethics committee to deal with thorny problems will give them a sense of security and added confidence that the facility will do the right thing.

THE ROLE OF ETHICS COMMITTEES IN POSTACUTE CARE

Long-Term Care

The emergence of the ethics committee in long-term care is a creative response to managed care and other external pressures. It can enable the clinical process to run more smoothly and at the same time it can develop systemic safeguards. The ability to frame issues in a way that encourages mutual understanding across institutional and community boundaries nurtures respect, which in turn leads to greater commonality of purpose.

Bringing outsiders into the inner workings of a long-term care facility is normally an anathema to the facility's administration. Therefore, the incentive to open the facility to outsiders must be greater than the fear of exposure.

Home Health Care

Home health providers are increasingly faced with the task of providing a certain level of care and at the same time are constrained by managed care contracts as well as Medicare/Medicaid provisions to provide that care at minimum cost. Since home health providers do not have the same supports as exist in many other health care settings and have to make decisions and exercise judgment on their own, they experience constraints and tradeoffs more acutely than many other caregivers. Often caught between a rock and a hard place, they need to develop a framework for addressing cost issues and to create formal mechanisms to prevent patient care from being compromised.

They also need to protect their patients and challenge inappropriate constraints without jeopardizing their relationships with managed care partners. One mechanism for achieving this is a community-based ethics committee. Often challenges to third-party payers are perceived negatively. The payers are inclined to view the providers as wanting to supply services ad infinitum and accordingly respond to most challenges as if they were unreasonable. A central forum for decision making may very well have greater credibility than any individual caregiver.

A committee with local representatives, including a community leader and local clergy, as well as representatives from local health care organizations can solve cost-constraint problems and repair negative images. It can also serve as a creative forum for addressing a wide range of patient care delivery and ethical issues.

Without policies, ethics ultimately boils down to individual opinions. While opinions have an important place in ethical discourse, they should be examined, tested, and graded and should always be held tentatively, and left open to revision.

To retain control of their destiny, care providers must deal with ethical issues proactively and on the basis of hard knowledge. The need to discover creative solutions to problems poses an exciting challenge to long-term care and home health providers.

THE INSTITUTIONAL ETHICS COMMITTEE

Establishing a framework for making decisions regarding ethical issues is an important step for a long-term care facility or home health agency to take. The fact that ethics committees are usually interdisciplinary testifies to the importance of diversity of perspective for handling a wide range of problems, many of them complex. For example, people often say they have an ethical problem they want to address when what they really mean is that they are concerned with legal liability. They disguise legal questions as ethical ones. This covering of one's backside mentality has been and will probably continue to be a significant motivating factor in bringing issues to the attention of an ethics committee, since this forum is more accessible and less threatening than the hospital legal counsel or an outside attorney.

One initial step is to identify why a given concern is brought to the attention of the committee and to sort out the legal, ethical, and administrative components. This serves several purposes: (1) it minimizes the scattergun approach to problem solving (the wider the spread, the greater chance of being on target); (2) it allows the committee to define precisely the issues at hand; (3) it can break down a complex problem into simpler components; and (4) it allows the committee to identify any confusions and misperceptions that exist.

What is discussed in the committee must be kept confidential. Talking in the elevator or the hallway about a case that is currently being considered is inappropriate. This is particularly true where sensitive concerns are voiced in the committee that would not have been voiced in a less protected setting.

Whether the problem at hand is primarily legal or ethical in nature, it must be addressed. The doctor and patient still must make a decision together. Or if the patient's wishes are unknown or unclear and there are no advance directives and no appropriate surrogate, the physician will have to act in the best interests of the patient.

Ethical committee discussions create an opportunity for enriched understanding and allow caregivers to deal with difficult problems better than in the past. They also can increase the comfort level of those involved in a decision-making situation and allow them to hold in abeyance their own moral preconceptions and prejudices and look at issues in a clearer way and without feeling threatened.

EDUCATIONAL TASKS

Educating Committee Members

An ethics committee must be provided with certain "tools of the trade." Members need to be familiar with key ethical and legal principles and how to define issues, test provisional decisions, and offer advice They need up-to-date materials and other resources. Developing a small library of books or articles is a sensible way of increasing members' knowledge and skills.

Although models can be used for developing policies, going through the process of development themselves is important for committee members so that they understand why the specific language was employed. Understanding this will help them perform their advisory role and reduce the chance of conflict. For example, if the committee chooses not to use the words "heroic measures" and replaces them with something more appropriate, the reason behind the choice is important, particularly when a caregiver approaches the committee for advice and uses "heroic measures" to define the issue. The committee hopefully will be able to explain that heroism implies sacrificing oneself or putting oneself in danger for a noble cause and that therefore "heroic measures" is inappropriate for referring to procedures that do no more than prolong the dying process. Being supplied with that insight might be extremely helpful to the staff member who has come to the committee for advice.

Educating Staff

If staff do not understand why a policy was created or changed or framed in the way it was, they likely will not take ownership of it, and the development of the policy will be little more than an interesting intellectual exercise on the part of the committee. The staff must receive in-service training on policies and procedures if they are to have a positive effect.

Occasionally an interesting case arises, a recurrent or even an unusual problem is identified, or a new regulation is put into place. These are appropriate teaching moments, and the ethics committee should use them as part of the process of educating staff about ethical issues and problem solving.

Educating Patients and the Community

Developing brochures, informing patients of options and resources available to them, and developing community education programs using outside consultants or committee members are all tasks that an ethics committee should perform or at least be involved with.

COMPOSITION OF THE COMMITTEE

As a general rule, an institutional ethics committee should have at least seven members but no more than ten, although many varieties involving substantially more or less than those suggested have been effective.. Obviously, the structure and membership of a particular committee will depend on what resources are available, whether the organization is part of an integrated delivery system, and whether it is a home health agency, long-term care facility, or some other kind of postacute care facility or agency.

The makeup of the committee will largely be determined by the assigned role, scope, and charge of the committee. For example, is the committee intended to play an educational, advisory, or decision-making role? Is it going to be a facility-based, shared or network model, or community-based committee?

Typical ethics committee members include the following:

- the director of nursing
- the medical director

- the head of the agency or facility
- the director of social work
- the director of pastoral care
- representatives from managed care and/or management company organizations (if appropriate)
- representatives from other community postacute care providers (e.g., long-term care facilities and home health agencies)
- representatives from referring institutions (e.g., hospitals and clinics)
- dietitians and other appropriate health professionals

CASE CONSULTATION

When a patient case is being considered, people with whom the patient has established a strong relationship, including those from previous stays at other facilities, should be considered for inclusion or at least contacted to obtain pertinent information. Also, people with special talents in the facility or agency can be integrated into the decision-making process. Insurance and risk management personnel are often appropriate advisors, and their participation can serve as an opportunity for committee members to learn how to address similar problems in the future.

Depending on the content of the case, other parties may be invited to attend special sessions. If, for example, the case concerns admission and transfer policies, representatives from the appropriate departments should be present.

People who face ethical and legal issues regularly or have experience dealing with such issues and are interested in serving on the ethics committee should be considered for membership. In smaller or rural facilities without a legal counsel, risk management and quality assurance personnel or a local attorney with interest in medical ethics would offer an important perspective on many issues likely to arise.

If the committee is to be primarily a policy-making group, there will be leaders and few if any doers. However, if clinical advising is part of the committee's charge, those responsible for care at the bedside must be included. Department heads may have clinical responsibilities, but they do not have the same perspective as staff nurses, for example, who must occasionally make on-the-spot decisions in the middle of the night.

The committee, whether or not its main job is developing and upgrading policies, will still have a responsibility to educate physicians, nurses, and other caregivers and support them when they are faced with difficult decisions.

CASE STUDIES

Case 1

When Mrs. J. entered a long-term care facility, ten years ago, she was aware it would not perform certain procedures or honor certain wishes, and she agreed to its terms. Now, however, she has become much sicker and is subject to sharp uncontrollable pain shooting into her limbs. She never envisioned spending the last days of her life in severe pain and she is adamant she does not want to be kept alive merely to suffer. She is becoming weak and, while she still has the capacity to make her wishes known, she clearly states that under no circumstances shall a feeding tube or even an IV be inserted to prolong her life. The facility says that it will not honor such a wish.

- What is the likely outcome of the dispute between Mrs. J. and the long-term care facility?
- Can patients give up the right to change their mind?

Suppose this long-term care facility originally had a policy of honoring patients' end-of-life wishes but has recently been purchased by a religious-oriented health care network and now will not honor certain wishes. When Mrs. W. entered the facility, she was told she could request a DNR order and it would be respected. Now, at the end of life and in extreme pain, she is told the facility's new policy does not permit the staff to abide by her wish to be allowed to die.

- What responsibilities does the facility have?
- What rights does Mrs. W. have?
- What role might a community ethics committee play in such a scenario?

- What role might an institutional ethics committee play in such a scenario?

Case 2

Mr. R., a resident of Dream Acres for nine years, has a fluctuating capacity to understand information. He has had a legal guardian for the past five years and has no surviving family members. He has developed a deteriorative disease for which there is no cure and has repeatedly indicated that he does not want any treatment for the disease. His guardian, on the other hand, demands that appropriate measures to control his symptoms and extend his life be undertaken. The guardian also informs the facility that should the resident suffer cardiac or pulmonary arrest, he must be resuscitated.

- What must be done if the patient suffers cardiac or pulmonary arrest?
- What if he refuses antibiotics or to take medicine for his condition?
- What role should the facility's policies regarding DNR, guardianship, and conflict resolution play in this type of situation?

REFERENCE

1. *Romona Osgood per Young, Brenda; Young, Chastity v. Genessee Regional Medical Center.* Genessee County Circuit Court, Michigan, filed January 25, 1994, decided March 1996. New hearing scheduled April 15, 1996. Case reported in *National Health Lawyers News Report*; 1996, March; 24(3):6.

11

The Community-Based Ethics Committee: A New Concept To Meet New Challenges

Whereas an institutional ethics committee may serve as a forum for conflict resolution as well as an important resource for education and advice, a community-based ethics committee can be used to tackle system-related issues, which in many ways are more complicated than intrafacility issues. It has the potential to prevent certain problems from arising by increasing consistency among different health care organizations and by shaping the way in which access, availability, and continuity issues are addressed.

The committee can also be a base for outreach into the community, and thus involving community leaders is an essential strategy.

Given the perception that making money is primary for them and patient care is secondary, long-term care institutions already have two strikes against them. Thus having some forum to increase their credibility, such as a community-based ethics committee, makes good sense. An ethics committee can also provide room for input and negotiation, which is a growing need, since pressures from managed care organizations are forcing clinicians and administrators to compromise the very thing they are expected to provide—care.

THE VOICE OF THE COMMUNITY

Managed care requires that provider organizations become integral partners in the attempt to supply high-quality services within cost constraints. Shared accountability and shared ownership are essential if the attempt is to succeed. A community-based ethics committee can assist in the functional integration of the members of a managed care network where it indeed becomes a network. The process may be time consuming at first, but the participants can anticipate and deal with issues that arise in an organized and coherent fashion, respond to what is good and what is bad, recommend modifications, and generally influence the way services are provided in the network.

If the committee is to serve as a voice to and for the community, its composition must reflect not only the mission of the various provider organizations but also the mandate to create a seamless delivery system. Case managers, social workers, residents' family members, acute care liaisons (physicians and nurses), clergy, and community leaders are appropriate members, as are intelligent and informed lawyers with both administrative and clinical sensitivity. The reason behind opening the ethics committee to the broader community is to get the community to understand the difficult life-determining issues routinely addressed by providers. Community representatives, by sharing responsibility and accountability in facing tough issues, will learn to respect the provider organizations and will be more inclined to act as their advocates in the community. Finally, having third-party payers participate in the ethics committee will create a tremendous opportunity to minimize misperceptions and bad blood and create a true continuum of care.

ENSURING CONTINUITY OF PATIENT WISHES

The need to resolve issues such as the coordination and continuity of patient wishes across provider organizations is reason enough to develop a community-based committee. For example, take the case of a terminally ill patient who no longer requires the intensity of care provided in a hospital and has been transferred back into the home with appropriate home care supports. The family, with the assistance and guidance of home health nurses and aides, serves as the primary support system for the patient. It was given the assurance that should the patient become too difficult to manage, she could be sent to a long-term care facility. This presents no problem so far, if coordination and planning allow for such mobility. The problem arises when other service agencies in the community get involved in the case.

PREVENTING FIRST RESPONDERS FROM RESUSCITATING AGAINST A PATIENT'S WISHES

Imagine a patient suffering from severely labored breathing. The emergency medical technicians (EMTs) are called in to help the patient and if necessary take the patient to the emergency department. These personnel often kick into high gear in the throes of an emergency. This is desirable so long as their intervention is consistent with the wishes of the patient. In this particular case, the family has asked the patient's physician to write a letter indicating the patient has a terminal condition and does not wish to avail herself of cardiopulmonary resuscitation. They produce this letter to the EMTs. The EMTs, however, are still uncomfortable. They are worried that if they fail to do everything they can, they may get sued or lose their licenses. At the same time, they became EMTs in order to help people, not to override people's wishes. Is that letter enough to rely on? What if the family members are just overwhelmed by the circumstances and are not thinking clearly? What if the cause of the distress is a mucous plug and the act of intubation could free the plug and easily avert death? Also, why did the family members call for support in the first place if they did not really want it?

Furthermore, the emergency department may legitimately be reluctant to accept the letter as an expression of the patient's current wishes. The letter was written when the patient was a resident of a long-term care facility. She has since returned home, and the change in settings may have caused her to change her mind. On top of that, the emergency department may hold the view that long-term care facilities do not employ the same rigor and safeguards in writing DNR orders as does their hospital.

Developing ways to reasonably and safely respond to individual requests, ensure consistency across institutional lines, and reduce fears on the part of the families and first responders is a worthy community goal. It is important to clarify obligations, protocols, policies, and procedures surrounding such issues, and an ethics committee composed of caregivers from various kinds of health care facilities can play a major role in such an endeavor.

SAFEGUARDING THE WISHES OF PATIENTS WHILE CLARIFYING THE OBLIGATIONS OF CAREGIVERS

In situations like the one described above, how can an ethics committee identify the most appropriate way to address the multiple needs without sacrificing the self-determination of patients or obstructing the professional duties of caregivers? In each case that comes before the committee, the committee's first step should be to examine

- the wishes of the patient
- the directive from the physician to the first responders
- the perceptions and responsibilities of the first responders
- the roles and responsibilities of the emergency personnel
- the role and status of family members

Everyone wants to do the right thing. No one wants to err by doing too little or too much. The first responders, who are unlikely to know the parties on the scene, have legitimate concerns. In fact, all the people involved have legitimate concerns, and a community-based committee can address those concerns and hopefully arrive at a reasonable solution that takes into account everyone's needs and wants.

First responders to an emergency as well as emergency department personnel are often frustrated and confused when dealing with a family that called for help but at the same time wants to restrict help. Getting beyond their frustration is a necessary step in solving the problem.

EMTs may perceive the family members as filled with denial or overwhelmed with grief, but they have a job to do. What is needed is a mechanism to ensure that patients' wishes are honored. One possible solution is a state-mandated "orange form," such as the one the state of Arizona uses. Each patient with a DNR order has a number that first responders can call to get the phone number of the appropriate hospital, home health agency, or long-term care facility, which can confirm the validity of the order.

Caregivers must deal more effectively with patient self-determination across the health care continuum. The health care delivery system will not become seamless magically. It is caregivers who need to repair the gaps—by developing better ways of coordinating services across traditional boundary lines.

In hospitals and nursing homes, when a new team begins its shift or changes its rotation, the transfer of critical patient information can be delayed or the information can even be lost. The problems of transmitting information from facility to facility are obviously more complex and require radical solutions. For example, why shouldn't there be community or interfacility DNR or transfer orders? Implementing a community-wide policy on end-of-life issues would help prevent aberrations in the provision of services and the infringement of patient rights. This is the sort of policy that community-based ethics committees are intended to concern themselves with.

MEMBERSHIP IN THE COMMUNITY-BASED ETHICS COMMITTEE

There are many issues that have a broad impact on the community, and the membership of a community-based ethics committee should reflect that fact. The membership should include locally influential people who can speak for the community and act as barometers of community concern. Enlisting community leaders can be of great value and make the committee much more effective. The committee itself will then be viewed as speaking for the community, and it will be more successful in addressing issues and topics of common importance and seeing them with a broad vision rather than from the limited perspective of a particular institution.

Having a political leader on the committee, perhaps even the mayor or a representative from the mayor's office, can be very helpful, particularly when bond issues or changes in the architecture of the system are required. Local clergy are often appropriate choices for membership, not necessarily because of their advanced training in ethics (which many do not have) but because they are trusted by their congregants and are often intimately involved in many of the complex and difficult situations families and patients face. They are aware of the impediments, frustrations, fears, and anxieties that their congregants experience and can act as their advocates in committee deliberations.

An attorney who is sensitive to community issues and knowledgeable about health care law would be a very valuable committee member. Cost is no deterrent, since community-based ethics committee members serve on a voluntary basis and without remuneration. Participation is perceived as a civic responsibility. It is important to get the right kind of lawyer—one who is filled with the spirit of cooperation—and avoid lawyers who constantly find fault and do little more than impede deliberation and decision making.

Trustees or key members of major health care organizations in the community can assist in identifying impediments and supports. So can key representatives of special interest groups. The best representatives are those who know the mission and have decision-making authority in the organizations they are representing.

An ethics consultant or a person with advanced training in ethics can be a helpful resource for training and education as well as for developing tools for analyzing problems and identifying solutions. If the ethicist has experience working with health care facilities, that is ideal. Knowing what has and has not been effective can save valuable time and can stimulate progress.

Those involved in liaison and triage functions and the movement of patients between institutions may be able to contribute important insights regarding issues related to these functions. Other possible committee members include EMTs, emergency department staff, and risk management and quality assurance personnel, local businesspeople, representatives of insurance companies and other third-party payers.

However, the committee should not be a Noah's ark, nor is there a recipe for determining its membership. If necessary, outside consultants and specialists can be used as resources so regular members should be chosen based on their status in the community, their talents, their position in key organizations, and their character.

A community-based ethics committee is not a viable substitute for an institutional ethics committee, as they have different roles. However, certain members of an institutional committee can and should serve on a community committee.

Generally, the community committee will deal with broader issues than the institutional committee. The community committee would generally review, not individual cases, but rather types of anticipated or recurrent cases that could be effectively addressed through its intervention. The only times a community committee would get involved in an individual case would be if the central issue was a recurrent one that could not be resolved at the institutional level. A family or patient might petition a community committee as a resource, but the committee would have the final decision as to whether to accept the case.

An institution can deal with ethical issues in a variety of ways: through meetings of an ethics committee but also through discussions during case management rounds, teaching rounds, or even special ethics rounds. For a community, a community-based ethics committee is virtually the only vehicle for confronting community-wide ethical issues. In addition, it is a wonderful forum for networking and developing jointly sponsored educational programs, and it can be an excellent barometer of concern about the health care system.

COORDINATION AND NETWORKING

The problems and issues the committee will likely address may not be complex but will require the imagination and creative energy of people with vision and a good overview of the community. Years ago, I was involved in creating a hospice program in Cambridge, Massachusetts, as part of a Harvard Community Health Outreach initiative. When the key players got together, they realized that they already had all the resources necessary to offer services needed in the community. It was merely a matter of knowing how to network among themselves and integrate existing health care, transportation, and volunteer services into a single package.

Although a community-based ethics committee is a superb resource for ethics-related networking, it is not the only resource. Liaisons with partners and sister organizations and other sectors of the health care community can set the stage for addressing a wide range of issues, ethical issues included.

OTHER ADVANTAGES OF COMMUNITY-BASED ETHICS COMMITTEES

A community-based ethics committee can become an advocate for the health care organizations represented on the committee as well as for the community. It can insulate the community from bad decision making and enhance its skills in dealing with issues that affect the community. It is a benevolent way to get people involved. A community network can create a community vision.

If anyone blows the whistle on a long-term care facility, it is likely to be an emergency department. One reason for different provider organizations to work together in an integrated multi-institutional setting is to develop a system for solving common problems and fostering the sharing of responsibilities and accountabilities.

Inconsistencies in policy can occur between departments in the same hospital, but inconsistencies between the hospital and a long-term facility are a virtual certainty and are sure to be much more pronounced. Furthermore, if discussions between and coordination of effort by the hospital emergency room and the long-term care facility have not occurred, advance directives and DNR orders may be viewed as spurious and not as an indication of the wishes of a patient who presents to the emergency department.

As mentioned above, a community-based ethics committee can also function as a marketing tool for creating private census. It creates an image of sharing rather than secrecy. In addition, provider organizations who are represented on the committee are seen as proactive leaders rather than as only responding to allegations of malpractice.

Long-term care facilities have an image problem and they can use a community-based ethics committee to polish their image. Home health agencies do not have the same problem. Their special need, because of the independence associated with home health care, is to make sure their policies and procedures are known by other types of provider organizations. Thus, a community-based ethics committee is a "natural" for home health, since it is a wonderful mechanism for identifying and creating linkages to the community and addressing continuity of care and continuity of consent concerns.

CASE STUDIES

Case 1

Mr. Z., after being in the hospital for 200 days, has become decisionally incompetent. His doctor says that he has never shared any information on how he would like to continue with his medical treatment. The nurses on staff patently disagree. They looked through the chart and found numerous notations of remarks made by Mr. Z. about what he wanted and what he did not want. They wonder if they should either highlight these notes or group them together in one inclusive progress note, with appropriate dates and times, in today's progress notes to stimulate the physician to honor the patient's wishes.

- What role might conflict resolution play?
- Is this a quality of care issue?
- Is this a risk management issue?
- Who is ultimately in charge of Mr. Z.'s care?

Case 2

A 46-year-old man is hospitalized with amyotrophic lateral sclerosis. He requires ventilatory support to increase his vital capacity but is reluctant to go on a ventilator. He says he does not want to become prisoner to a machine. He has clearly indicated that he didn't want to become another Karen Ann Quinlan. His physician tells him that if he does not go on the ventilator he will surely die. The physician also assures him that if the patient determines enough is enough or the physician feels there is no benefit, there will be no problem removing the ventilator. The physician has checked with the hospital legal counsel, who agrees with the physician's position. The patient reluctantly allows the physician to intubate him and put him on the ventilator on the strict condition that he be taken off when he decides he wants to be taken off.

Several months later, after being discharged home, the patient is still receiving ventilatory support but is in a much more deteriorative state. He feels that the burden now outweighs the benefits, and he decides to exercise his right to choose and have the ventilator withdrawn. The physician calls the hospital legal counsel, who advises her that since the patient is no longer in the hospital, the promise made to him could not be honored with the hospital's blessing. The attorney admits to being uncertain about the physician's and hospital's liability outside of the hospital setting.

- On whom should the patient rely for help in this situation?
- Who is responsible for the patient?
- What is the ethical thing to do and why?
- What role might a community-based ethics committee play?
- What responsibility does the physician who provided him assurances have?
- What responsibility does the hospital and its legal counsel have?

12

Integrating Clinical, Legal, Ethical, and Administrative Problem Solving and Decision Making

EXPANDING THE NOTION OF WHO CAN DECIDE

A particular case with which I was involved was complicated by the fact that the patient was unwilling to be approached directly about his wishes regarding various medical options and was comfortable handing decision-making authority to his wife—a woman from whom he had been divorced for 15 years. This type of situation occasionally arises. A patient has a strong bond of trust with someone but has not gone through the process of formally making that person his or her health care surrogate or durable agent. For example, it is not uncommon for older people to meet and move in together but refrain from marrying so as to maximize their social security benefits. Partners in such relationships are not easily accommodated under the guidelines determining who can decide in the absence of a clearly expressed advance directive.

Criteria as to who counts in end-of-life decision making need to be clarified, and standards of evidence for substituted judgment need to be unpacked. This is not a minor issue in terms of numbers and specific populations at risk for having their wishes ignored. Indeed, the numbers of such people are increasing and some solution is desperately needed. Part of the solution would undoubtedly be to ensure "continuity of consent" and view consent as a dynamic process rather than as a discrete event.

CONTINUITY OF CONSENT: TOWARD A SEAMLESS DELIVERY SYSTEM

Establishing consent should involve creating a baseline using information about the patient's wishes from former hospitalizations, nursing home stays, primary care physicians, clergy, home health personnel, and family members. Agreement between past expressions of wishes by the patient and information from the chart can be critically important. One valuable tactic is to have the patient fill out a supplement to the admissions form that indicates whether the patient has a designated spokesperson (and, if so, the name of the individual), a living will, or a durable power of attorney for health care (Exhibit 12-1).

Clear information about the patient's wishes can increase physician comfort and diminish conflict and uncertainty. In a family conference or pastoral care conference, it can keep the participants on track and make it likely the patient's wishes will actually be honored. It can even be used to protect a patient from a third party who, because of unresolved grief or some other agenda, might try to compromise decision making by seeking legal guardianship.

When a resident is transferred from a long-term care facility to a hospital, critical information about the resident's wishes is often not transmitted to the new health care team. It seems so strange that such information—information that may prevent family members or caregivers from undermining the resident's self-determination—is not transferred right along with the resident.

Similarly, why is such information not transmitted to home health caregivers? Hospital staff, working with a patient and family, may spend enormous energy in conflict resolution, patient care, pastoral care, family conferences, ethics committee deliberations, and the like and yet, when the patient is transferred to the home or another facility, may make no attempt to share the information gleaned or the significant content of the discussions. Failure to pass on such information breaks the continuity of consent and can result in unwanted procedures being performed. Indeed, it may well constitute negligence and be legally actionable.

REVIEW AND SUMMARY

This book provides resources for addressing a wide range of ethical and legal issues in diverse settings, developing new ethics-related policies and procedures, and educating staff, patients, and families about such policies and issues. It offers

Exhibit 12–1 Sample Admissions Form Supplement

Your wishes will help shape your care. To better serve you, we require certain information upon admission.

Name _____

        Last   First   Middle   (Nickname)

Address_____

        Street   City   State

Phone _____

        Home   Work

If you become unable to express yourself, who do you designate as your spokesperson for purposes of medical decision making:

Name _____

        Last   First   Middle   (Nickname)

Address_____

        Street   City   State

Phone _____

        Home   Work

Relationship _____

Do you already have a legally designated spokesperson?

Yes _____   No _____

Do you have a living will?

Yes _____   No _____

Do you have a durable power of attorney?

Yes _____   No _____

Known allergies or precautions:

_____

Do you suffer from a deteriorative, degenerative, or terminal disease?

Yes _____   No _____

Have you indicated any specific wishes regarding treatment to your doctor or other caregiver?

_____

guidance on how to use ethics rounds and institutional and community-based ethics committees; explores the concept of patient autonomy and its implications for policy development, documentation, and risk management; and recommends ways to insulate against legal liability.

Most health care professionals do not possess the tools to address ethical and legal issues. Even those who have had the benefit of a survey course in ethics do not possess the necessary technical skills to define an ethical issue, break it down into simple components, and deal with these individually. The purpose of this book is to teach health care professionals how to frame issues, use decision-making models, evaluate alternative decisions and solutions to problems, and justify their positions using the principles of autonomy, truth telling, and professional responsibility, among others.

The importance of going beyond institutional walls to network with other provider organizations has been emphasized. Such networking can include developing or participating in a community-based ethics committee. This type of committee has certain advantages; an institutional ethics committee and ethics rounds each have others. Consideration should be given to all three problem-solving fora.

Because of the pressures of managed care—rationing, gatekeeping, and cost constraints—caregivers must expend additional energy to advocate for or support those who fall under their care and to ensure their wishes are respected. Knowing what their professional duties, including their ethical responsibilities, actually are allows caregivers to determine where they need to take a stand and where they can try to work with payers to resolve issues and problems.

The word *professional* comes from the Latin word *profiteri*, meaning "to avow publicly." A professional professes to have something distinctive to offer. A health care professional professes to be able to offer medical assistance to people who are sick or hurt, and thus are especially vulnerable. Because they are dealing with people who are vulnerable, caregivers are in a position of extreme power, which they can either use wisely or abuse. They have the authority to decide whether patients have decisional capacity and can thus afford or deny them the right to choose. What keeps caregivers from misusing their power is their professional integrity and their understanding of their legal and ethical responsibilities.

Many people are still afraid to avail themselves of health care. In fact, as people get older, they often develop an increased fear of medical settings and are worried that their wishes will be compromised. Therefore, it is very important that provider organizations have some forum for discussing and resolving ethical issues so as to ensure that patients are treated with maximum respect and are given the opportunity to refuse or avail themselves of medical services if that is their true desire. One helpful tool for supporting patients' self-determination is a brochure or pamphlet that describes the range of advance directives and surrogate designations available for use (Exhibit 12-2.)

Ethics can be a positive force for change. Learning how to deal with legal and ethical issues will reshape the way health professionals provide care. Ethical deliberation can clarify what obligations caregivers have to those they serve. I believe that by developing better tools to address ethical issues and justify their decisions, caregivers will become more supportive of their patients and be able to meet the challenges that they will face in the near and distant future. It is hoped that the exposure to understanding pivotal legal and ethical principles will demythologize what are perceived to be impossible and insurmountable issues and allow caregivers to face and address ethical challenges of the future.

Exhibit 12-2 Brochure on Advance Directives and Surrogacy

YOUR WISHES ARE IMPORTANT IN SHAPING YOUR CARE

MAKING HEALTH CARE DECISIONS

We want to provide you with information and support regarding advance directives as you make health care decisions. An "advance directive" tells us what your wishes are regarding medical treatment if you become unable to tell us yourself. This brochure will help you as you think about your choices, help you to know what to discuss with your doctor and family, and explains your right to participate in making decisions. It also tells you how, under this hospital's policies and procedures, to continue to make decisions if you become unable to personally make them.

HOW WILL DECISIONS BE MADE IF YOU ARE UNABLE TO DECIDE FOR YOURSELF?

An adult patient never loses the right to make treatment decisions when he becomes incapacitated. However, in circumstances where sickness or mental state interferes with your ability to make decisions, questions arise as to who can act for you and how this person knows or decides what to do. Under our policies, we first look for written answers from three sources: (1) an agent appointed through a *medical durable power of attorney* or *health care surrogate* designation (which is not as flexible as the durable power of attorney), that is, someone you have appointed in writing to act in your behalf; (2) a *living will*, that is, a document stating what you want or don't want done if you are terminally ill (and "terminally" is extremely narrowly defined); or (3) *legal guardianship*. Guardianship is often imposed rather than chosen. The guardian may not know what your wishes are or be able to honor or enforce them. It is better to choose someone you trust while you have the capacity to do so. Unfortunately, not everyone has gone through the formalities of a written document, that is, a directive indicating in advance what your directions or wishes are or who you want as your spokesperson, or has a court-appointed guardian. When a patient has not provided the hospital with directions in writing, our policies have us consider information and

---

continues

Exhibit 12-2 continued

viewpoints, including your past oral statements, that is, things you said to friends, family, or clergy, or other information provided by family or friends about your wishes, and any instructions from you, to get a reasonable indication of your wishes.

TYPES OF ADVANCE DIRECTIVES

A durable power of attorney, as well as the health care surrogate, allows you to name or designate an "agent" or "surrogate" who can make medical treatment decisions if you become unable to make them yourself. The health care surrogate is much more restrictive than the durable power of attorney and may not assure your wishes to the same degree. The durable power of attorney generally becomes effective when you no longer possess the capacity to participate in medical decision making. The durable power of attorney is much less restrictive than other advance directives and often is the best formal way to ensure your wishes. Not all advance directives require that you consult an attorney, although you may do so if you wish.

HOW WILL THE FACILITY KNOW IF YOU HAVE ANY ADVANCE DIRECTIVES?

We will ask you when you are being admitted here whether you have designated in writing specific directions or a specific person by some form of advance directive regarding your medical care. If you have, we will file the documents that you give us in your medical record at the hospital, including the name, address, and telephone numbers of the person who you would like to make decisions for you in the event you are no longer able to make them for yourself.

HOW CAN YOU MAKE AN ADVANCE DIRECTIVE THROUGH A DURABLE POWER OF ATTORNEY FOR HEALTH CARE, DESIGNATE A HEALTH CARE SURROGATE, OR CREATE A LIVING WILL?

Many advisors in the health care field believe that the durable power of attorney is an excellent way to have your wishes known because it allows you to appoint someone whom you trust to act and speak for you. The health care surrogate designation can also be helpful but is more restrictive

continues

Exhibit 12-2 continued

than the durable power of attorney. If you wish to further explore this option, we will be glad to have a representative assist you.

Another written directive is the living will. Unlike a health care surrogate designation or medical durable power of attorney, a living will does not name anyone to make decisions for you and does not possess the flexibility of other advance directives. Instead, it lists or describes the kinds of medical treatments you wish to have or do not wish to have if you become terminally ill (it is very restrictive in its definition of terminal illness).

WILL YOUR WISHES BE HONORED IF YOU HAVE NO ADVANCE DIRECTIVE?

There is no law that says you have to make an advance directive. Our policies recognize that many patients have had discussions about their wishes involving medical treatment options with their family, clergy, and close friends, even if they have not written them down. Most often this information is helpful and reliable enough for us to be able to honor your wishes.

HOW CAN YOU GET MORE INFORMATION?

For additional information, you may contact the Social Services Office at ext. ____ to assist you with any other questions regarding advance directives or any other item covered in this brochure. This is part of our ongoing commitment to better serve you. If you want more detailed information about relevant state law, we recommend you consult your attorney.

CASE STUDIES

Case 1

Mr. B. has inoperable colorectal cancer. He is 89 years old and has lived at home with assistance for over 10 years. He has long complained of pain but the family and his caregivers have not always taken his complaints seriously. He is somewhat cranky and has always loved to make a fuss. The pain issue has been addressed many times and the response has usually been the same: keep him on what he is already taking.

Mr. B.'s pain, however, has now become more pronounced, and his physician has prescribed a strong analgesic to relieve the pain, a morphine-based pill administered by mouth. The medication is given in small doses so as not to compromise his respiration. The physician tells the home health aide to administer one pill every 6 hours but to double the dosage if it does not work. After taking a single pill, Mr. B. goes to sleep, but when he awakens, he still complains of pain. The home health aide feels that a second pill might compromise respiration and kill him and is very reluctant to give it to him. She calls into the agency for support, and a nurse comes to the scene and discovers that the patient is becoming septic.

- What should the aide do?
- What should the nurse do?
- Should prognosis play a significant role in determining whether to give the second dose?
- Does the patient's wish not to be in pain influence whether the second dose should be administered?
- What are the main ethical issues in this case?

Case 2

[This is a variation of an earlier case. It is included here so that the reader can address the issues anew after learning about ethics committees and problem-solving techniques.]

Mr. G. was hospitalized after he was discovered to have lung cancer. Surgery revealed that his cancer had metastasized to the brain. Soon after admission, he began to throw fits. He would lie on the floor of the main corridor, flail his arms and legs, and scream. These fits ended when a supportive and trusting relationship was formed between Mr. G. and the hospital's hospice team. The regimen he is under neither prescribes treatments contrary to his wishes nor constitutes abandonment and neglect. Mr. G. now seems at peace with himself, has come to terms with his imminent death, and wants very much to spend the remainder of his life at home with his wife.

However, a serious problem exists. Mr. G.'s wife pretends to want him sent home when she is in his presence, but when she leaves the room she begs the physician to keep her husband in the hospital. She claims that his being at home is too physically and psychologically burdensome for her. Amidst this conflict arises still another problem: nothing more can be done for Mr. G. medically, and so the hospital utilization review committee will recommend that he be discharged to a lower level of care when next it meets. Since his wife does not want him to come home and there are no other supports available, he will likely be sent to a nursing home. If the nursing home is unable to minister to his emotional and psychological needs, which is a distinct possibility, rapid deterioration in his emotional state is inevitable.

The attending physician thinks Mr. G. will survive only for another week or so. He knows that if he lies a little, omits certain information from the chart or concocts false notes, he may be able to keep Mr. G. in the hospital. He could also informally ask the social services department to be less aggressive in finding a lower-level bed for Mr. G., but in doing so he risks undermining the trust of third-party payers. He feels a transfer would be medically counterproductive and emotionally harmful. He also feels that not doing whatever he can to provide care for this patient would be a violation of his professional and ethical responsibility and constitute abandonment. The problems he faces are not medical ones but problems caused by cost containment.

- What responsibilities does the physician have?
- What responsibilities do other caregivers have?
- Can the caregivers ethically support the wife's dishonesty?
- Should the patient be told of his wife's real wishes?
- Could a hospice program provide the supports necessary to solve this problem?
- Are there administrative ways to address this issue?

This case gives rise to some complex ethical questions. Many of them center around the issue of lying. Mrs. G. disguises her inability to care for her husband at home by pretending to want him sent home as soon as possible. The staff are then placed in the position of having to lie, at least if they want to ensure Mr. G. is well taken care of and not learn of his wife's distress. This raises a question as to whom the staff, including the physician, have their main responsibility—the patient or the family. Many physicians consider shielding the patient from unnecessary stress to be an important part of their care. On the other hand the wife's denial may be necessary for her phychological well-being as she struggles to come to terms with her husband's impending death. However, as an advocate for his patient, the physician might at least approach the wife to try to determine whether she could deal with a confrontation over the issue of home care. Perhaps an appropriate referral could be made to a hospice group that offers both medical and emotional support. Deciding what to do in such situations is not a matter of applying a decision-making template. The principles must be blended with the concrete reality that confronts those who must decide.

Topical Bibliography

Lora A. Robbins, MS, LS, MS, HSA
Loyola University Medical Center Library
Maywood, Illinois

This topical bibliography is intended as a user-friendly resource of readily available materials to assist the researcher/student. It is arranged by subject categories with the major focus on home health and/or long-term care.

GENERAL

AMA Council on Ethical and Judicial Affairs. Ethical issues in managed care. *JAMA*. 1995;273(4):330–335.

Annas GJ. Do feeding tubes have more rights than patients? *Hastings Cent Rep*. 1986;16:26–28.

Mill JS. *Utilitarianism*. Indianapolis, Ind: Hackett Publishing Co, Inc; 1979.

Rando TA. *Grief, Dying and Death: Clinical Interventions for Caregivers*. Champaign, Ill: Research Press; 1984.

Reiser S, Dyck A, Curran W. *Ethics in Medicine: Historical Perspectives and Contemporary Concerns*. Cambridge, Mass: MIT Press; 1977.

Robbins DA. Cost containment and terminal care: an essay into the ethics of appropriateness. *Long Term Care Adm*. 1981;9:41–47.

Robbins DA. *Ethical Dimensions of Clinical Medicine*. Springfield, Ill: Charles C Thomas, Publisher; 1981.

Robbins DA. *Legal and Ethical Issues in Cancer Care in the United States*. Springfield, Ill: Charles C Thomas, Publisher; 1983.

Robbins DA. Update: The removal of life supports in long-term care facilities. *J Long Term Care Adm*. 1985;13:3–5.

Robbins DA. Legal and ethical dilemmas in emergency care. *Emergency Medical Services*. 1987;16:19–21.

Robbins DA. Edge of life. Advance directive protocols and the Patient Self Determination Act. *Kentucky Hospitals Magazine*. 1992;9:26–27.

ADVANCE DIRECTIVES AND LIVING WILLS

Adams JG, Derse AR, Gotthold WE, Mitchell JM, Moskop JC, Sanders AB. Ethical aspects of resuscitation. *Ann Emerg Med.* 1992;21:1273–1276.

Ahronheim J, Weber D. *Final Passages: Positive Choices for the Dying and Their Loved Ones.* New York, NY: Simon & Schuster, Inc; 1992.

Bliss MR. Resources, the family and voluntary euthanasia. *Br J Gen Pract.* 1990;40(332):117–122.

Brown LM, Rousseau GK. Resuscitation status begins at home. *Am J Nurs.* 1990;4:24–26.

Carr P. Implications of the implementation of the Patient Self-Determination Act for nurses in the field. *Home Healthcare Nurse.* 1992;10:53–54.

Cassel CK, Hays JR, Lynn J. Alzheimer's: decisions in terminal care. *Patient Care.* 1991;25(18):125–137.

Coll PP, Anderson D. Advanced directives for homebound patients. *J Am Board Fam Pract.* 1992;5:359–360. Letter; comment.

Cummings NB. Social, ethical, and legal issues involved in chronic maintenance dialysis. In: Maher JF, ed. *Replacement of Renal Function by Dialysis.* 3rd ed. Boston: Kluwer Acad; 1989:1141–1158.

Daly MP, Sobal J. Advance directives among patients in a house call program. *J Am Board Fam Pract.* 1992;5:11–15. Comments.

Dorff EN. "A time to be born and a time to die": a Jewish medical directive for health care. *United Synagogue Review.* 1992;45:20–22.

Ethical considerations in resuscitation. *JAMA.* 1992;16:2282–2288.

Ethical issues of resuscitation. American College of Emergency Physicians. *Ann Emerg Med.* 1992;21:1277.

Freedman M. Helping home bound elderly clients understand and use advance directives. *Soc Work Health Care.* 1994;20:61–73.

Fried TR, Gillick MR. Medical decision-making in the last six months of life: choices about limitation of care. *J Am Geriatr Soc.* 1994;42:303–307.

Garson KB. Do not resuscitate options in home care. *Home Healthcare Nurse.* 1992;10:21–23.

Gillick MR. *Choosing Medical Care in Old Age: What Kind, How Much, When To Stop.* Cambridge, Mass: Harvard University Press; 1994.

Guidelines for cardiopulmonary resuscitation and emergency cardiac care. Emergency Cardiac Care Committee and Subcommittees, American Heart Association. Part VIII. Ethical considerations in resuscitation. *JAMA.* 1992;16:2282–2288. Comments.

Havlir D, Brown L, Rousseau GK. Do not resuscitate discussions in a hospital-based home care program. *J Am Geriatr Soc.* 1989;1:52–54.

High DM. Surrogate decision making. Who will make decisions for me when I can't? *Clin Geriatr Med.* 1994;10:445–462. Review.

Holly CM. Advance directives: a program design for home healthcare. *Home Healthcare Nurse.* 1993;11:34–38.

Hudson T. Advance directives: still problematic for providers. *Hosp Health Network.* 1994;68:46.

Iserson KV. Foregoing prehospital care: should ambulance staff always resuscitate? *J Med Ethics.* 1991;17:19–24.

Iserson KV. The "no code" tattoo—an ethical dilemma. *West J Med.* 1992;156:309–312.

Iserson KV, Rouse F. Prehospital DNR orders. *Hastings Cent Rep.* 1989;19:17–19. Case study and commentaries.

Jecker NS, Schneiderman LJ. Medical futility: the duty not to treat. *Camb Q Healthcare Ethics.* 1993;2:151–159.

Kapp MB. Legal and ethical issues in family caregiving and the role of public policy. *Home Health Care Serv Q.* 1991;12:5–28.

Kapp MB. *Geriatrics and the Law: Patient Rights and Professional Responsibilities.* 2nd ed. New York, NY: Springer Publishing Co, Inc; 1992.

Kellogg FR, Crain M, Corwin J, Brickner PW. Life-sustaining interventions in frail elderly persons. Talking about choices. *Arch Intern Med.* 1992;152:2317–2320.

Key ethical issues in palliative care: evidence to House of Lords Select Committee on Medical Ethics. 1993. The Council, London, England.

Klem CB. Attitudes of direct care staff in home healthcare toward advance directives. *Home Healthcare Nurse.* 1994;12:55–59.

Krynski MD, Tymchuk AJ, Ouslander JG. How informed can consent be? New light on comprehension among elderly people making decisions about enteral tube feeding. *Gerontologist.* 1994;34:36–43.

Loewy EH. Advance directives and surrogate laws. Ethical instruments or moral cop-out? *Arch Intern Med.* 1992;152:1973–1976.

Loewy EH. Limiting but not abandoning treatment in severely mentally impaired patients: a troubling issue for ethics consultants and ethics committees. *Camb Q Healthcare Ethics.* 1994;3:216–225.

Lynn J. Ethical issues in caring for elderly residents of nursing homes. *Prim Care.* 1986;13:295–306.

Mahoney J, Singer PA, Lowy FH, Hilberman M, Mitchell A, Stroud CE, et al. Cost savings at the end of life. *N Engl J Med.* 1994;331:477–478. Letters and response.

Markson LJ, Steel K. Using advance directives in the home-care setting. *Generations.* 1990;14:25–28.

Markson LJ, Fanale J, Steel K, Kern D, Annas G. Implementing advance directives in the primary care setting. *Arch Intern Med.* 1994;154:2321–2327. Comments.

Meier DE, Cassel CK. Nursing home placement and the demented patient: a case presentation and ethical analysis. *Ann Intern Med.* 1986;1:98–105.

Miles SH. Advanced directives to limit treatment: the need for portability. *J Am Geriatr Soc.* 1987;1:74–76. Editorial.

Minogue B, Reagan JE. Can complex legislation solve our end-of-life problems? *Camb Q Healthcare Ethics.* 1994;3:115–124.

Murphy DJ. Improving advance directives for healthy older people. *J Am Geriatr Soc.* 1990;38:1251–1256.

Olson E, Chichin E, Meyers H, Schulman E, Brennan F. Early experiences of an ethics consult team. *J Am Geriatr Soc.* 1994;42:437–441. Comments.

Osman H, Perlin TM. Patient self-determination and the artificial prolongation of life. *Health Soc Work.* 1994;19:245–252.

Outerbridge DE, Hersh AR. *Easing the Passage: A Guide for Prearranging and Ensuring a Pain-Free and Tranquil Death via a Living Will, Personal Medical Mandate, and Other Medical, Legal, and Ethical Resources.* New York, N.Y.: HarperCollins; 1991.

Reisner A. Instructions for the Valley of the Shadow: a medical directive (living will). *United Synagogue Review.* 1992;44:22–23.

Robbins DA. Edge of life. Advance directive protocols and the Patient Self Determination Act. *Kentucky Hospitals Magazine.* 1992;9:26–27.

Schneiderman LJ, Kaplan RM, Pearlman RA, Teetzel H. Do physicians' own preferences for life-sustaining treatment influence their perceptions of patients' preferences? *J Clin Ethics.* 1993;4:28–33.

Scitovsky A, Capron AM. Medical care at the end of life: the interaction of economics and ethics. In: Breslow L, Fielding JE, Lave LB, eds. *Annual Review of Public Health.* Palo Alto, CA: Annual Reviews; 1994:75.

Sharp JW, Roncagli T. Home parenteral nutrition in advanced cancer: ethical and psychosocial aspects. *Cancer Pract.* 1993;1:119–124.

Terry M, Zweig S. Prevalence of advance directives and do-not-resuscitate orders in community nursing facilities. *Arch Fam Med.* 1994;3:141–145.

Thomasma DC. Advance directives and health care for the elderly. In: Hackler C, Moseley R, Vawter DE, eds. *Advance Directives in Medicine.* New York, N.Y.: Praeger Pubs; 1989:93–109.

Thomasma DC. Models of the doctor-patient relationship and the ethics committee: part two. *Camb Q Healthcare Ethics.* 1994;3:10–26.

Turner JF, Mason T, Anderson D, Gulati A, Sbarbaro JA. Physicians' ethical responsibilities under co-pay insurance: should potential fiscal liability become part of informed consent? *J Clin Ethics.* 1995;6:68–72.

Van Bommel H. *Choices: For People Who Have a Terminal Illness, Their Families, and Their Caregivers.* Port Washington, NY: NC Press; 1986.

Ventres W, Nichter M, Reed R, Frankel R. Limitation of medical care: an ethnographic analysis. *J Clin Ethics.* 1993;4:134–145. Comments.

Wanzer SH. The physician's responsibility toward hopelessly ill patients: a second look. *N Engl J Med.* 1989;320:844–849.

Waymack MH, Taler GA. *Medical Ethics and the Elderly: A Case Book.* Chicago, Ill: Pluribus Press, Inc; 1988.

Wenger NS, Halpern J. The physician's role in completing advance directives: ensuring patients' capacity to make healthcare decisions in advance. *J Clin Ethics.* 1994;5:320–323. Comments.

Wicclair MR. *Ethics and the Elderly.* New York, NY: Oxford University Press; 1993.

COMMUNITY NURSING AND AFTERCARE

Barkauskas VH. Case management within home care: old ideas and new themes. *Home Healthcare Nurse.* 1994;12:8. Editorial.

Bertolotti G, Carone M. From mechanical ventilation to home-care: the psychological approach. *Monaldi Arch Chest Dis.* 1994;49:537–540.

Burger AM, Erlen JA, Tesone L. Factors influencing ethical decision making in the home setting. *Home Healthcare Nurse.* 1992;10:16–20.

Jenkins HM. Ethical dimensions of leadership in community health nursing. *J Community Health Nurs.* 1989;6:103–112.

Kimaid Y, Votava KM, Myers E. Patient advocacy: one agency's positive results with the administrative law judge process. *Home Healthcare Nurse.* 1994;12:29–32.

Klem CB. Attitudes of direct care staff in home healthcare toward advance directives. *Home Healthcare Nurse.* 1994;12:55–59.

Kristoff B, Selin S, Miller MP. Patients' rights and ethical dilemmas in home care: incorporation of psychological concepts. *Home Healthcare Nurse.* 1994;12:45–50. Published erratum appears in *Home Healthcare Nurse;* 1994;12:8.

Power-Smith P, Evans M. Dementia. Communal confusion. *Nurs Times.* 1993;89:26–28.

Rozell BR, Newman KL. Extending a critical path for patients who are ventilator dependent: nursing case management in the home setting. *Home Healthcare Nurse.* 1994;12:21–25.

EMERGENCY MEDICAL SERVICES

Ethical considerations in resuscitation. *JAMA.* 1992;16:2282–2288.

Iserson KV. Foregoing prehospital care: should ambulance staff always resuscitate? *J Med Ethics.* 1991;17:19–24.

Iserson KV, Rouse F. Prehospital DNR orders. *Hastings Cent Rep.* 1989;19:17–19. Case study and commentaries.

Koenig KL, Haynes B. Prehospital "do-not-resuscitate" orders—a new option. *West J Med.* 1993;159:602–603.

Miles SH. Advanced directives to limit treatment: the need for portability. *J Am Geriatr Soc.* 1987;1:74–76. Editorial.

Robbins DA. Legal and ethical dilemmas in emergency care. *Emergency Medical Services.* 1987;16:19–21.

END-OF-LIFE DECISION MAKING

Gelman D, Springen K. The doctor's suicide van. *Newsweek,* June 18, 1990; 46–49.

Guidelines on the Termination of Life-Sustaining Treatment and the Care of the Dying: A Report by the Hastings Center. Briarcliff Manor, N.Y.: Hastings Center; 1987.

Joint Report of the Council on Ethical and Judicial Affairs and the Council on Scientific Affairs: Persistent vegetative state and the decision to withdraw or withhold life support. *Proceedings of the House of Delegates of the AMA.* June 1989; 314–316.

Kass LR. Neither for love nor money: why doctors must not kill. *Public Interest.* 1969;94:25–46.

Lynn J, Childress JF. Must patients always be given food and water? *Hastings Cent Rep.* October 1983;17–21.

Office of Technology Assessment Task Force. *Life-Sustaining Technologies and the Elderly.* Philadelphia: Science Information Resource Center; 1988.

President's Commission for the Study of Ethical Problems in Medicine and Biomedical and Behavioral Research. *Deciding to Forego Life-Sustaining Treatment: A Report on the Ethical, Medical and Legal Issues in Treatment Decisions.* Washington, D.C.: Government Printing Office, 1987.

Quill TE. Death and dignity: a case of individualized decision making. *N Engl J Med.* 1991;324:691–694.

Report B of the Council on Ethical and Judicial Affairs: Do not resuscitate orders. *Proceedings of the House of Delegates of the AMA.* December 1987; 170–171.

Report C of the Council on Ethical and Judicial Affairs: Euthanasia. *Proceedings of the House of Delegates of the AMA.* June 1988; 258–260.

Report D of the Council on Ethical and Judicial Affairs: Guidelines for the appropriate use of do-not-resuscitate orders. *Proceedings of the House of Delegates of the AMA.* December 1990; 180–185.

Sprung CL. Changing attitudes and practices in foregoing life-sustaining treatment. *JAMA.* 1990;263:2211–2215.

Washington state doctors trying for alternative to euthanasia ballot. *AM News.* February 11, 1991; 3, 46.

ETHICS COMMITTEE

Abel E. Ethics committees in home health agencies. *Public Health Nurs.* 1990;7:256–259.

Anderson B, Hall B. Parents' perceptions of decision making for children. *J Law Med Ethics.* 1995;23:15–19.

Burger AM, Erlen JA, Tesone L. Factors influencing ethical decision making in the home setting. *Home Healthcare Nurse.* 1992;10:16–20.

Cassel CK. Ethical issues in the conduct of research in long term care. *Gerontologist.* 1988;3(suppl):90–96.

Curtin LL. DNR in the OR: ethical concerns and hospital policies. *Nurs Manage.* 1994;25:29–31.

Edinger W. Expanding opportunities for ethics committees: residential centers for the mentally retarded and developmentally disabled. *Camb Q Healthcare Ethics.* 1994;3:226–232.

Edwards BS. When the physician won't give up. *Am J Nurs.* 1993;93:34–37.

Edwards BS. When the family can't let go. *Am J Nurs.* 1994;94:52–56.

Ethical considerations in resuscitation. *JAMA.* 1992;16:2282–2288.

Haddad AM, Kapp MB. *Ethical and Legal Issues in Home Health Care: Case Studies and Analyses.* Norwalk, Conn: Appleton & Lange; 1991.

Howe EG. Attributing preferences and violating neutrality. *J Clin Ethics.* 1992;3:171–175. Comment.

Hudson T. Are futile-care policies the answer? Providers struggle with decisions for patients near the end of life. *Hosp Health Network.* 1994;68:26–30.

Jecker NS, Schneiderman LJ. Medical futility: the duty not to treat. *Camb Q Healthcare Ethics.* 1993;2:151–159.

Kanoti GA. Writing a proposal for determining patient decisional capacity. *HEC* [Hospital Ethics Committee] *Forum.* 1994;6:12–17.

Kapp MB. *Geriatrics and the Law: Patient Rights and Professional Responsibilities.* 2nd ed. New York, NY: Springer Publishing Co, Inc; 1992.

Keffer MJ, Keffer HL. U.S. ethics committee: perceived versus actual roles. *HEC Forum.* 1991;3:227–230.

Loewy EH. Suffering as a consideration in ethical decision making. *Camb Q Healthcare Ethics.* 1992;1:135–142.

Loewy EH. Limiting but not abandoning treatment in severely mentally impaired patients: a troubling issue for ethics consultants and ethics committees. *Camb Q Healthcare Ethics.* 1994;3:216–225.

Milholland DK. Privacy and confidentiality of patient information. Challenges for nursing. *J Nurs Adm.* 1994;24:19–24.

Minogue B, Reagan JE. Can complex legislation solve our end-of-life problems? *Camb Q Healthcare Ethics.* 1994;3:115–124.

Orlowski JP. The HEC and conflicts of interest in the health care environment. *HEC Forum.* 1994;6:3–11.

Price DM. Forgoing treatment in an adult with no apparent treatment preference: a case report. *Theor Med.* 1994;15:53–60.

Ross JW, Glaser JW, Rasinski-Gregory D, Gibson JM, Bayley C. *Health Care Ethics Committees: The Next Generation.* Chicago, Ill: American Hospital Publishing, Inc; 1993.

Rubin S, Zoloth-Dorfman L. First-person plural: community and method in ethics consultation. *J Clin Ethics.* 1994;5:49–54. Editorial; comment.

Schwartz RL. Autonomy, futility, and the limits of medicine. *Camb Q Healthcare Ethics.* 1992;1:159–164.

Snyder JW, Swartz MS. Deciding to terminate treatment: a practical guide for physicians. *J Crit Care.* 1993;8:177–185.

Teel KW. From Quinlan to today. *Camb Q Healthcare Ethics.* 1992;1:291–294.

Thomasma DC. Models of the doctor-patient relationship and the ethics committee: part two. *Camb Q Healthcare Ethics.* 1994;3:10–26.

Waymack MH, Taler GA. *Medical Ethics and the Elderly: A Case Book.* Chicago, Ill: Pluribus Press, Inc; 1988.

Young PA, Pelaez M. The in-service education program of the Home Health Assembly of New Jersey. *Generations.* 1990;14:37–38.

HEALTH CARE POLICY AND REFORM

Abel PE. Ethics committees in home health agencies. *Public Health Nurs.* 1990;7(4):256–259.

Adams JG, Arnold R, Siminoff L, Wolfson AB. Ethical conflicts in the prehospital setting. *Ann Emerg Med.* 1992;21:1259–1265.

Annas GJ. Will the real bioethics (commission) please stand up? *Hastings Cent Rep.* 1994;24:19–21.

Arno PS, Bonuck KA, Padgug R. The economic impact of high-technology home care. *Hastings Cent Rep.* 1994;24(5):S15–S19.

Aroskar MA. Research in community-based care of persons with AIDS: an ethical framework. In: Community-Based Care of Persons with AIDS: Developing a Research Agenda 1990. *AHCPR Conference Proceedings.* Minneapolis, 15–16 Aug 1989. U.S. Agency for Health Care Policy and Research, Rockville, MD 1990, A:127–131.

Aroskar MA. Decisions at the end of life: an ecological view. In: Hodges LW, ed. *Social Responsibility: Business, Journalism, Law, Medicine.* Lexington, VA; 1993:56–68.

Arras JD. The technological tether: an introduction to ethical and social issues in high-tech home care [and] executive summary of project conclusions. *Hastings Cent Rep.* 1994;24(suppl):S1–S3.

Barkauskas VH. Case management within home care: old ideas and new themes. *Home Healthcare Nurse.* 1994;12:8. Editorial.

Binstock RH. Long-term care for older people: moral and political challenges of access. In: Monagle JF, Thomasma DC, eds. *Health Care Ethics: Critical Issues.* Gaithersburg, MD: Aspen Publishers; 1994:158–167.

Blanchette PL. Age-based rationing of health care. *Hawaii Med J.* 1995;54:507–509.

Bliss MR. Resources, the family and voluntary euthanasia. *Br J Gen Pract.* 1990;40(332):117–122.

Blumenfield S, Lowe JI. A template for analyzing ethical dilemmas in discharge planning. *Health Soc Work.* 1987;12:47–56.

Bovbjerg R, Held PJ, Diamond LH. Provider-patient relations and treatment choice in the era of fiscal incentives: the case of the End-Stage Renal Disease Program. *Milbank Q.* 1987;2:177–202.

Chadwick R, Russell J. Hospital discharge of frail elderly people: social and ethical considerations in the discharge decision-making process. *Aging & Society.* 1989;9:277–295.

Charlesworth M, Gifford S. *The Place of Ethics in Health Care Resource Allocation: Where to Now?* Canberra, Australia: National Health and Medical Research Council; 1992.

Collette J, Windt PY, Jahnigen DW. Medical decision-making, dying, and quality of life among the elderly. In: Smeeding TM, et al., eds. *Should Medical Care be Rationed by Age?* Totowa, NJ: Rowman & Littlefield; 1987:99–118.

Collopy B, Dubler N, Zuckerman C. The ethics of home care: autonomy and accommodation. *Hastings Cent Rep.* 1990;20(2)(suppl):S1–S16.

Cummings NB. Social, ethical, and legal issues involved in chronic maintenance dialysis. In: Maher JF, ed. *Replacement of Renal Function by Dialysis.* 3rd ed. Boston: Kluwer Acad; 1989:1141–1158.

Dubler N. Individual advocacy as a governing principle. *J Case Manage.* 1992; 1:82–86.

Edelstein H, Lang A. Posthospital care for older people: a collaborative solution. *Gerontologist.* 1991;31:267–270.

Estes CL. Cost containment and the elderly: conflict or challenge? *J Am Geriatr Soc.* 1988;1:65–72.

Ethical considerations in resuscitation. *JAMA.* 1992;16:2282–2288.

Feldman C, Olberding L, Shortridge L, Toole K, Zappin P. Decision making in case management of home healthcare clients. *J Nurs Adm.* 1993;23:33–38.

Forrow L, Daniels N, Sabin JE. When is home care medically necessary? *Hastings Cent Rep.* 1991;21(4):36–38.

Fry ST. Ethical issues in total parenteral nutrition. *Nutrition.* 1990;6:329–332.

Gatter RA Jr, Moskop JC. From futility to triage. *J Med Philos.* 1995;20:191–205.

Gillick MR. *Choosing Medical Care in Old Age: What Kind, How Much, When to Stop.* Cambridge, Mass: Harvard University Press; 1994.

Iserson KV. Foregoing prehospital care: should ambulance staff always resuscitate? *J Med Ethics.* 1991;17:19–24.

Jenkins HM. Ethical dimensions of leadership in community health nursing. *J Community Health Nurs.* 1989;6:103–112.

Jennings B, Callahan D, Caplan AL. Ethical challenges of chronic illness. *Hastings Cent Rep.* 1988;18(1)(suppl):S1–S16.

Johnson JE. Nurses vs doctors: the battle between the caregivers in health care reform. *Nursing Connections.* 1994;7:1–3.

Kane RA, Caplan AL. *Ethical Conflicts in the Management of Home Care: The Case Manager's Dilemma.* New York, NY: Springer Publishing Co, Inc; 1993.

Kapp MB. Are risk management and health care ethics compatible? *Perspect Healthcare Risk Manage.* 1991;11:2–7.

Kapp MB. Legal and ethical issues in family caregiving and the role of public policy. *Home Health Care Serv Q.* 1991;12:5–28.

Kerschner PA. Assuring access to long-term care: legal, ethical, and other barriers. In: Kapp MB, Pies HE, Doudera A, Edward BS, eds. *Legal and Ethical Aspects of Health Care for the Elderly.* Ann Arbor, MI: Health Administration Press; 1986:24–36.

Koop CE. Families caring for disabled need long-term support. *Health Progress.* 1986;67(6):52–54.

Luce JM. Physicians do not have a responsibility to provide futile or unreasonable care if a patient or family insists. *Crit Care Med.* 1995;23:760–766. Comments.

Lumsdon K. Crash course: piecing together the continuum of care. *Hosp Health Network.* 1994;68:26–28.

Lynn J. Ethical issues in caring for elderly residents of nursing homes. *Prim Care.* 1986;13:295–306.

MacMillan-Scattergood D. Ethical conflicts in a prospective payment home health environment. *Nurs Economics.* 1986;4:165–170.

McEwen M. Promoting interdisciplinary collaboration. *Nurs Health Care.* 1994;15:304–307.

Meier DE, Cassel CK. Nursing home placement and the demented patient: a case presentation and ethical analysis. *Ann Intern Med.* 1986;1:98–105.

Oppenheimer EA. Decision-making in the respiratory care of amyotrophic lateral sclerosis: should home mechanical ventilation be used? *Palliat Med.* 1993;7(suppl):49–64.

Paris NM, Hines J. Payer and provider relationships: the key to reshaping health care delivery. *Nurs Adm Q.* 1995;19:13–17.

Post SG. Justice, community dialogue, and health care. *J Soc Philos.* 1992;23:23–34.

Rozell BR, Newman KL. Extending a critical path for patients who are ventilator dependent: nursing case management in the home setting. *Home Healthcare Nurse.* 1994;12:21–25.

Schwartzberg JG, Stein-Hulin J. Home health care: surmounting the obstacles to Medicare coverage. *Geriatrics.* 1991;46:28–30.

Scitovsky A, Capron AM. Medical care at the end of life: the interaction of economics and ethics. In: Breslow L, Fielding JE, Lave LB, eds. *Annual Review of Public Health.* Palo Alto, CA: Annual Reviews; 1994:75.

Sharp JW, Roncagli T. Home parenteral nutrition in advanced cancer: ethical and psychosocial aspects. *Cancer Pract.* 1993;1:119–124.

Stoltzfus DP, Stamatos JM. An appraisal of the ethical issues involved in high-technology cancer pain relief. *J Clin Ethics.* 1991;2:113–115. Commentary.

Taylor RM, Lantos JD. The politics of medical futility. *Issues Law Med.* 1995;11:3–12.

Thomasma DC. Advance directives and health care for the elderly. In: Hackler C, Moseley R, Vawter DE, eds. *Advance Directives in Medicine.* New York, NY: Praeger; 1989:93–109.

Wanzer SH. The physician's responsibility toward hopelessly ill patients: a second look. *N Engl J Med.* 1989;320:844–849.

Waymack MH, Taler GA. *Medical Ethics and the Elderly: A Case Book.* Chicago, Ill: Pluribus Press, Inc; 1988.

Weindling AM. Ethics and economics of health care. Prognosis, a traditional alternative to futility. *BMJ.* 1995;310:1671–1672. Letter.

Whiting M. Issues in community care. In: Brykczynska GM, ed. *Ethics in Paediatric Nursing.* London: Chapman and Hall; 1989:65–80.

Wicclair MR. *Ethics and the Elderly.* New York, NY: Oxford University Press; 1993.

Young PA, Pelaez M. The in-service education program of the Home Health Assembly of New Jersey. *Generations.* 1990;14:37–38.

INFORMED CONSENT

Adams JG, Arnold R, Siminoff L, Wolfson AB. Ethical conflicts in the prehospital setting. *Ann Emerg Med.* 1992;21:1259–1265.

Agich GJ. Reassessing autonomy in long-term care. *Hastings Cent Rep.* 1990;20:12–17.

Agich GJ. *Autonomy and Long-Term Care.* New York, NY: Oxford University Press; 1993.

Ahronheim J, Weber D. *Final Passages: Positive Choices for the Dying and Their Loved Ones.* New York, NY: Simon & Schuster, Inc; 1992.

Arras JD, Dubler NN. Bringing the hospital home. Ethical and social implications of high-tech home care. *Hastings Cent Rep.* 1994;24(suppl):S19–S28.

Block JA. Evaluating the patient's capacity for making decisions. In: Dunkle RE, Wykle ML, eds. *Decision Making in Long-Term Care: Factors in Planning.* New York, NY: Springer Publishing Co, Inc; 1988:31–39.

Brock DW. Decisionmaking competence and risk. *Bioethics.* 1991;5:105–112.

Cassel CK. Ethical issues in the conduct of research in long term care. *Gerontologist.* 1988;3(suppl):90–96.

Cassel CK, Hays JR, Lynn J. Alzheimer's: decisions in terminal care. *Patient Care.* 1991;25(18):125–137.

Cohen CA, Meslin EM, Shulman KI. Dementia at home: ethical issues and clinical realities. In: Berg JM, Karlinsky H, Lowy FH, eds. *Alzheimer's: Disease Research: Ethical and Legal Issues.* Toronto: Carswell; 1991: 317–330.

Cummings NB. Social, ethical, and legal issues involved in chronic maintenance dialysis. In: Maher JF, ed. *Replacement of Renal Function by Dialysis* 3rd ed. Boston: Kluwer Acad; 1989:1141–1158.

Ethical considerations in resuscitation. *JAMA.* 1992;16:2282–2288.

Ferrara PJ. Expanding autonomy of the elderly in home health care programs. *New England Law Review.* 1990;25:421–455.

Fins J. Encountering diversity: medical ethics and pluralism. *Journal of Religion & Health.* 1994;33:23–27.

Fry ST. Ethical issues in total parenteral nutrition. *Nutrition.* 1990;6:329–332.

Gillick MR. *Choosing Medical Care in Old Age: What Kind, How Much, When to Stop.* Cambridge, Mass: Harvard University Press; 1994.

Groome PA, Hutchinson TA, Tousignant P. Content of a decision analysis for treatment choice in end-stage renal disease: who should be consulted? *Med Decis Making.* 1994;14:91–97.

Haddad AM, Kapp MB. *Ethical and Legal Issues in Home Health Care: Case Studies and Analyses.* Norwalk, Conn: Appleton & Lange; 1991.

Hofland BF. Autonomy in long term care: background issues and a programmatic response. *Gerontologist.* 1988;3(suppl):3–9.

Igoe S, Cascella S, Stockdale K. Ethics in the OR: DNR and patient autonomy. *Nurs Manage.* 1993;24:112A.

Iserson KV. Foregoing prehospital care: should ambulance staff always resuscitate? *J Med Ethics.* 1991;17:19–24.

Kanoti GA. Writing a proposal for determining patient decisional capacity. *HEC Forum.* 1994;6:12–17.

Kapp MB. Legal and ethical issues in family caregiving and the role of public policy. *Home Health Care Serv Q.* 1991;12:5–28.

Kapp MB. *Geriatrics and the Law: Patient Rights and Professional Responsibilities.* 2nd ed. New York, NY: Springer Publishing Co, Inc; 1992.

Kapp MB. Who's the parent here? The family's impact on the autonomy of older persons. *Emory Law Journal.* 1992;41:773–803.

Key ethical issues in palliative care: evidence to House of Lords Select Committee on Medical Ethics. 1993. The Council, London, England.

Kopelman LM. Conceptual and moral disputes about futile and useful treatments. *J Med Philos.* 1995;20:109–121.

Krynski MD, Tymchuk AJ, Ouslander JG. How informed can consent be? New light on comprehension among elderly people making decisions about enteral tube feeding. *Gerontologist.* 1994;34:36–43.

Loewy EH. Suffering as a consideration in ethical decision making. *Camb Q Healthcare Ethics.* 1992;1:135–142.

Lynn J. Ethical issues in caring for elderly residents of nursing homes. *Prim Care.* 1986;13:295–306.

Markson LJ, Steel K. Using advance directives in the home-care setting. *Generations.* 1990;14:25–28.

Meier DE, Cassel CK. Nursing home placement and the demented patient: a case presentation and ethical analysis. *Ann Intern Med.* 1986;1:98–105.

Murphy DJ. Improving advance directives for healthy older people. *J Am Geriatr Soc.* 1990;38:1251–1256.

National Hospice Organization. *Do-Not-Resuscitate (DNR) Decisions in the Context of Hospice Care.* Arlington, Va: National Hospice Organization; 1992.

Outerbridge DE, Hersh AR. *Easing the Passage: A Guide for Prearranging and Ensuring a Pain-Free and Tranquil Death via a Living Will, Personal Medical Mandate, and Other Medical, Legal, and Ethical Resources.* New York, NY: HarperCollins; 1991.

Schiedermayer D. *Putting the Soul Back in Medicine: Reflections on Compassion and Ethics.* Grand Rapids, Mich: Baker Books; 1994.

Smith ML. Futile medical treatment and patient consent. *Cleve Clin J Med.* 1993;60:151–154. Review.

Stoltzfus DP, Stamatos JM. An appraisal of the ethical issues involved in high-technology cancer pain relief. *J Clin Ethics.* 1991;2:113–115. Commentary.

Teres D. Trends from the United States with end of life decisions in the intensive care unit. *Intensive Care Med.* 1993;19:316–322. Review.

Turner JF, Mason T, Anderson D, Gulati A, Sbarbaro JA. Physicians' ethical responsibilities under co-pay insurance: should potential fiscal liability become part of informed consent? *J Clin Ethics.* 1995;6:68–72.

Ventres W, Nichter M, Reed R, Frankel R. Limitation of medical care: an ethnographic analysis. *J Clin Ethics.* 1993;4:134–145. Comments.

Wicclair MR. *Ethics and the Elderly.* New York, NY: Oxford University Press; 1993.

MEDICAL FUTILITY

Alpers A, Lo B. When is CPR futile? *JAMA.* 1995;273:156–158. Editorial; comment.

Anderson B, Hall B. Parents' perceptions of decision making for children. *J Law Med Ethics.* 1995;23:15–19.

Annas GJ. Do feeding tubes have more rights than patients? *Hastings Cent Rep.* 1986;16:26–28.

Asch DA, Hansen-Flaschen J, Lanken PN. Decisions to limit or continue life-sustaining treatment by critical care physicians in the United States: conflicts between physicians' practices and patients' wishes. *Am J Respir Crit Care Med.* 1995;151(pt 1):288–292. Comments.

Blanchette PL. Age-based rationing of health care. *Hawaii Med J.* 1995;54:507–509.

Brody BA, Halevy A. Is futility a futile concept? *J Med Philos.* 1995;20:123–144.

Capron AM. Medical futility: strike two. *Hastings Cent Rep.* 1994;24:42–43.

Caswell D, Cryer HG. Case study: when the nurse and physician don't agree. *J Cardiovasc Nurs.* 1995;9:30–42.

Curtis JR, Park DR, Krone MR, Pearlman RA. Use of the medical futility rationale in do-not-attempt-resuscitation orders. *JAMA.* 1995;273:124–128. Comments.

Ebell MH. When everything is too much. Quantitative approaches to the issue of futility. *Arch Fam Med.* 1995;4:352–356. Comments.

Ethical considerations in resuscitation. *JAMA.* 1992;16:2282–2288.

Gatter RA Jr, Moskop JC. From futility to triage. *J Med Philos*. 1995;20:191–205.

Griener GG. The physician's authority to withhold futile treatment. *J Med Philos*. 1995;20:207–224.

Hargrove MD Jr. A five-step approach to settling a dispute over futile care. *J La State Med Soc*. 1994;146:439–440.

Jecker NS, Schneiderman LJ. Medical futility: the duty not to treat. *Camb Q Healthcare Ethics*. 1993;2:151–159.

Jecker NS, Schneiderman LJ. Judging medical futility: an ethical analysis of medical power and responsibility. *Camb Q Healthcare Ethics*. 1995;4:23–35.

Jecker NS, Schneiderman LJ. When families request that "everything possible" be done. *J Med Philos*. 1995;20:145–163.

Key ethical issues in palliative care: evidence to House of Lords Select Committee on Medical Ethics. 1993: The Council, London, England.

Kopelman LM. Conceptual and moral disputes about futile and useful treatments. *J Med Philos*. 1995;20:109–121.

Leibson CM. The role of the courts in terminating life-sustaining medical treatment. *Issues Law Med*. 1995;10:437–451.

Luce JM. Physicians do not have a responsibility to provide futile or unreasonable care if a patient or family insists. *Crit Care Med*. 1995;23:760–766. Comments.

Mahoney J, Singer PA, Lowy FH, Hilberman M, Mitchell A, Stroud CE, et al. Cost savings at the end of life. *N Engl J Med*. 1994;331:477–478. Letters and response.

Marsden AK, Ng GA, Dalziel K, Cobbe SM. When is it futile for ambulance personnel to initiate cardiopulmonary resuscitation? *BMJ*. 1995;311:49–51.

Miller FG. The good death, virtue, and physician-assisted death: an examination of the hospice way of death. *Camb Q Healthcare Ethics*. 1995;4:92–97.

Nazarko L. A time to die: ethics of prolonging life. *Elder Care*. 1995;7:10.

Noland LR. HealthCare Ethics Forum '94: medical futility: a bedside perspective. *Clin Issues*. 1994;5:366–368.

Pronger L, Fehr T, Poulter-Friesen P, Powell L, Whytehead C, Wasylak T. Discontinuation of lifesupport. *Can Nurse*. 1995;91:51–53.

Robbins DA. Cost containment and terminal care: an essay into the ethics of appropriateness. *J Long Term Care Adm*. 1981;9:41–47.

Sade RM. Medical futility and ineffective care: a proposal for hospital policy. *J S C Med Assoc.* 1995;91:63–65.

Schiedermayer D. *Putting the Soul Back in Medicine: Reflections on Compassion and Ethics.* Grand Rapids, Mich: Baker Books; 1994.

Sharp JW, Roncagli T. Home parenteral nutrition in advanced cancer: ethical and psychosocial aspects. *Cancer Pract.* 1993;1:119–124.

Shaw AB. Acts of commission, omission, and demission or pulling the plug. *J R Soc Med.* 1995;88:18–19.

Sprung CL, Eidelman LA, Steinberg A. Is the physician's duty to the individual patient or to society? *Crit Care Med.* 1995;23:618–620. Editorial; comment.

Taylor RM, Lantos JD. The politics of medical futility. *Issues Law Med.* 1995;11:3–12.

Teno JM, Murphy D, Lynn J, Tosteson A, Desbiens N, Connors AF Jr, et al. Prognosis-based futility guidelines: does anyone win? SUPPORT Investigators. Study to Understand Prognoses and Preferences for Outcomes and Risks of Treatment. *J Am Geriatr Soc.* 1994;42:1202–1207.

Tong R. Towards a just, courageous, and honest resolution of the futility debate. *J Med Philos.* 1995;20:165–189.

Turner JF, Mason T, Anderson D, Gulati A, Sbarbaro JA. Physicians' ethical responsibilities under co-pay insurance: should potential fiscal liability become part of informed consent? *J Clin Ethics.* 1995;6:68–72.

Waisel DB, Truog RD. The cardiopulmonary resuscitation-not-indicated order: futility revisited. *Ann Intern Med.* 1995;122:304–308.

Weindling AM. Ethics and economics of health care. Prognosis, a traditional alternative to futility. *BMJ.* 1995;310:1671–1672. Letter.

Welk TA. Life-support and end-of-life questions: treatment or intervention? *J Intraven Nurs.* 1995;18:191–197.

Wicclair MR. *Ethics and the Elderly.* New York, NY: Oxford University Press; 1993.

MEDICAL TECHNOLOGY

Ahronheim J, Weber D. *Final Passages: Positive Choices for the Dying and Their Loved Ones.* New York, NY: Simon & Schuster, Inc; 1992.

Arras JD. The technological tether: an introduction to ethical and social issues in high-tech home care [and] executive summary of project conclusions. *Hastings Cent Rep.* 1994;24(5)(suppl):S1–S3.

Arras JD, Dubler NN. Bringing the hospital home. Ethical and social implications of high-tech home care. *Hastings Cent Rep.* 1994; 24 (suppl):S19–S28.

Brummel-Smith K. Home health care: how long will it remain "low tech"? *Southern California Law Review.* 1991;65:491–502.

Charlesworth M, Gifford S. *The Place of Ethics in Health Care Resource Allocation: Where to Now?* Canberra, Australia: National Health and Medical Research Council; 1992.

Dorff EN. "A time to be born and a time to die"; a Jewish medical directive for health care. *United Synagogue Review.* 1992;45:20–22.

Ferrell BR, Rhiner M. High-tech comfort: ethical issues in cancer pain management for the 1990s. *J Clin Ethics.* 1991;2:108–112.

Fry ST. Ethical issues in total parenteral nutrition. *Nutrition.* 1990;6:329–332.

Gillick MR. *Choosing Medical Care in Old Age: What Kind, How Much, When to Stop.* Cambridge, Mass: Harvard University Press; 1994.

Kaufman J. Case management services for children with special health care needs. A family-centered approach. *J Case Manage.* 1992;1:53–56.

Mahoney J, Singer PA, Lowy FH, Hilberman M, Mitchell A, Stroud CE, et al. Cost savings at the end of life. *N Engl J Med.* 1994;331:477–478. Letters and response.

Noddings N. Moral obligation or moral support for high-tech home care? *Hastings Cent Rep.* 1994;24(5)(suppl):S6–S10.

Outerbridge DE, Hersh AR. *Easing the Passage: A Guide for Prearranging and Ensuring a Pain-Free and Tranquil Death via a Living Will, Personal Medical Mandate, and Other Medical, Legal, and Ethical Resources.* New York, NY: HarperCollins; 1991.

Post SG. Justice, community dialogue, and health care. *J Soc Philos.* 1992;23:23–34.

Reisner A. Instructions for the Valley of the Shadow: a medical directive (living will). *United Synagogue Review.* 1992;44:22–23.

Schiedermayer D. *Putting the Soul Back in Medicine: Reflections on Compassion and Ethics.* Grand Rapids, Mich: Baker Books; 1994.

Scitovsky AA, Capron AM. Medical care at the end of the life: the interaction of economics and ethics. In: Breslow L, Fielding JE, Lave LB, eds. *Annual Review of Public Health.* Palo Alto, CA: Annual Reviews; 1994:75.

Stoltzfus DP, Stamatos JM. An appraisal of the ethical issues involved in high-technology cancer pain relief. *J Clin Ethics.* 1991;2:113–115. Commentary.

Thomasma DC. Advance directives and health care for the elderly. In: Hackler C, Moseley R, Vawter DE, eds. *Advance Directives in Medicine*. New York, NY: Praeger; 1989:93–109. 1994:i–109.

MENTAL COMPETENCY AND CAPACITY

Adams JG, Arnold R, Siminoff L, Wolfson AB. Ethical conflicts in the prehospital setting. *Ann Emerg Med*. 1992;21:1259–1265.

Agich GJ. *Autonomy and Long-Term Care*. New York, NY: Oxford University Press; 1993.

Block JA. Evaluating the patient's capacity for making decisions. In: Dunkle RE, Wykle ML, eds. *Decision Making in Long-Term Care: Factors in Planning*. New York, NY: Springer Publishing Co, Inc; 1988:31–39.

Brock DW. Decisionmaking competence and risk. *Bioethics*. 1991;5:105–112.

Cassel CK. Ethical issues in the conduct of research in long term care. *Gerontologist*. 1988;3(suppl):90–96.

Cassel CK, Hays JR, Lynn J. Alzheimer's: decisions in terminal care. *Patient Care*. 1991;25(18):125–127.

Chadwick R, Russell J. Hospital discharge of frail elderly people: social and ethical considerations in the discharge decision-making process. *Aging & Society*. 1989;9:277–295.

Cohen CA, Meslin EM, Shulman KI. Dementia at home: ethical issues and clinical realities. In: Berg JM, Karlinsky H, Lowy FH, eds. *Alzheimer's: Disease Research: Ethical and Legal Issues*. Toronto: Carswell; 1991: 317–330.

Cohen ES. The elderly mystique impediment to advocacy and empowerment. *Generations*. 1990;14:13–16.

Collopy BJ. Ethical dimensions of autonomy in long-term care. *Generations*. 1990;14:9–12.

Cummings NB. Social, ethical, and legal issues involved in chronic maintenance dialysis. In: Maher JF, ed. *Replacement of Renal Function by Dialysis*. 3rd ed. Boston: Kluwer Acad; 1989:1141–1158.

Downes BR. Guardianship for people with severe mental retardation: consent for urgently needed treatment. *Health Soc Work*. 1992;17:13–15.

Dubler NN. Improving the discharge planning process: distinguishing between coercion and choice. *Gerontologist*. 1988;3(suppl):76–81.

Ferrara PJ. Expanding autonomy of the elderly in home health care programs. *New England Law Review*. 1990;25:421–455.

Haddad AM, Kapp MB. *Ethical and Legal Issues in Home Health Care: Case Studies and Analyses.* Norwalk, Conn: Appleton & Lange; 1991.

High DM. Surrogate decision making. Who will make decisions for me when I can't? *Clin Geriatr Med.* 1994;10:445–462. Review.

Hofland BF. Autonomy in long term care: background issues and a programmatic response. *Gerontologist.* 1988;3(suppl):3–9.

Iserson KV. Foregoing prehospital care: should ambulance staff always resuscitate? *J Med Ethics.* 1991;17:19–24.

Kane RA, Caplan AL. *Ethical Conflicts in the Management of Home Care: The Case Manager's Dilemma.* New York, NY: Springer Publishing Co, Inc; 1993.

Kanoti GA. Writing a proposal for determining patient decisional capacity. *HEC Forum.* 1994;6:12–17.

Kapp MB. Legal and ethical issues in family caregiving and the role of public policy. *Home Health Care Serv Q.* 1991;12:5–28.

Kapp MB. *Geriatrics and the Law: Patient Rights and Professional Responsibilities.* 2nd ed. New York, NY: Springer Publishing Co, Inc; 1992.

Kapp MB. Who's the parent here? The family's impact on the autonomy of older persons. *Emory Law Journal.* 1992;41:773–803.

Key ethical issues in palliative care: evidence to House of Lords Select Committee on Medical Ethics. 1993. The Council, London, England.

Krynski MD, Tymchuk AJ, Ouslander JG. How informed can consent be? New light on comprehension among elderly people making decisions about enteral tube feeding. *Gerontologist.* 1994;34:36–43.

Lynn J. Ethical issues in caring for elderly residents of nursing homes. *Prim Care.* 1986;13:295–306.

Milholland DK. Privacy and confidentiality of patient information. Challenges for nursing. *J Nurs Adm.* 1994;24:19–24.

National Hospice Organization. *Do-Not-Resuscitation (DNR) Decisions in the Context of Hospice Care.* Arlington, Va: National Hospice Organization; 1992.

Olson E, Chichin E, Meyers H, Schulman E, Brennan F. Early experiences of an ethics consult team. *J Am Geriatr Soc.* 1994;42:437–441. Comments.

Osman H, Perlin TM. Patient self-determination and the artificial prolongation of life. *Health Soc Work.* 1994;19:245–252.

Outerbridge DE, Hersh AR. *Easing the Passage: A Guide for Prearranging and Ensuring a Pain-Free and Tranquil Death via a Living Will, Personal Medical Mandate, and Other Medical, Legal, and Ethical Resources,* New York, NY: HarperCollins; 1991.

Schiedermayer D. *Putting the Soul Back in Medicine: Reflections on Compassion and Ethics.* Grand Rapids, Mich: Baker Books; 1994.

Snyder JW, Swartz MS. Deciding to terminate treatment: a practical guide for physicians. *J Crit Care.* 1993;8:177–185.

Waymack MH, Taler GA. *Medical Ethics and the Elderly: A Case Book.* Chicago, Ill: Pluribus Press, Inc; 1988.

Weiler K, Helms LB, Buckwalter KC. A comparative study: guardianship petitions for adults and elder adults. *J Gerontol Nurs.* 1993;19:15–25.

Wicclair MR. *Ethics and the Elderly.* New York, NY: Oxford University Press; 1993.

Young A, Pignatello CH, Taylor MB. Who's the boss? Ethical conflicts in home care. *Health Progress.* 1988;11:59–62.

NURSING ETHICS

Barkauskas VH. Case management within home care: old ideas and new themes. *Home Healthcare Nurse.* 1994;12:8. Editorial.

Bertolotti G, Carone M. From mechanical ventilation to home-care: the psychological approach. *Monaldi Arch Chest Dis.* 1994;49:537–540.

Burger AM, Erlen JA, Tesone L. Factors influencing ethical decision making in the home setting. *Home Healthcare Nurse.* 1992;10:16–20.

Forrow L, Daniels N, Sabin JE. When is home care medically necessary? *Hastings Cent Rep.* 191;21(4):36–38.

Hogstel MO, Nelson M. Anticipation and early detection can reduce bowel elimination complications. *Geriatr Nurs.* 1992;13:28–33.

Jenkins HM. Ethical dimensions of leadership in community health nursing. *J Community Health Nurs.* 1989;6:103–112.

Kimaid Y, Votava KM, Myers E. Patient advocacy: one agency's positive results with the administrative law judge process. *Home Healthcare Nurse.* 1994;12:29–32.

Klem CB. Attitudes of direct care staff in home healthcare toward advance directives. *Home Healthcare Nurse.* 1994;12:55–59.

Kristoff B, Sellin S, Miller MP. Patients' rights and ethical dilemmas in home care: incorporation of psychological concepts. *Home Healthcare Nurse.* 1994;12:45–50. Published erratum appears in *Home Healthcare Nurse;* 1994; 12:8.

Muego C. Dying at home. *Nursing BC.* 1992;24:22–26.

Power-Smith P, Evans M. Dementia. Communal confusion. *Nurs Times.* 1993;89:26–28.

Rozell BR, Newman KL. Extending a critical path for patients who are ventilator dependent: nursing case management in the home setting. *Home Healthcare Nurse.* 1994;12:21–25.

Ruddick W. Transforming homes and hospitals. *Hastings Cent Rep.* 1994; 24(5)(suppl):S11–S14.

PATIENT ADVOCACY AND LEGAL GUARDIANS

Agich GJ. Reassessing autonomy in long-term care. *Hastings Cent Rep.* 1990;20:12–17.

Aroskar MA. Community health nurses: their most significant decision-making problems. *Nurs Clin North Am.* 1989;24:967–975.

Aroskar MA. Decisions at the end of life: an ecological view. In: Hodges LW, ed. *Social Responsibility: Business, Journalism, Law, Medicine.* 1993:56–68.

Batey JM, Horton AM. Homecare. The future is now. *ASHA.* 1992;34:45–47.

Berlin RM, Canaan A. A family systems approach to competency evaluations in the elderly. *Psychosomatics.* 1991;32:349–354.

Bigler BR. Critical care nursing: expanding roles and responsibilities within the community. *Crit Care Nurs Clin North Am.* 1990;2(3):493–502.

Binstock RH. Long-term care for older people: moral and political challenges of access. In: Monagle JF, Thomasma DC, eds. *Health Care Ethics: Critical Issues.* Gaithersburg, MD: Aspen Publishers; 1994:158–167.

Brock DW. Deciding for others: surrogate decision making for incompetent adults. *R I Med J.* 1991;74:105–111.

Capron AM. Medical futility: strike two. *Hastings Cent Rep.* 1994;24:42–43.

Carr P. Implications of the implementation of the Patient Self-Determination Act for nurses in the field. *Home Healthcare Nurse.* 1992;10:53–54.

Chadwick R, Russell J. Hospital discharge of frail elderly people: social and ethical considerations in the discharge decision-making process. *Ageing & Society.* 1989;9:277–295.

Chubon SJ. Ethical dilemmas encountered by home care nurses: caring for patients with acquired immune deficiency syndrome. *Home Healthcare Nurse.* 1994;12:12–17. Published erratum appears in *Home Healthcare Nurse,* 1994;12:8.

Cohen ES. The elderly mystique: impediment to advocacy and empowerment. *Generations.* 1990;14:13–16.

Dubler NN. Improving the discharge planning process: distinguishing between coercion and choice. *Gerontologist.* 1988;3(suppl):76–81.

Dubler NN. Individual advocacy as a governing principle. *J Case Manage.* 1992;1(3):82–86.

Edwards BS. When the physician won't give up. *Am J Nurs.* 1993;93:34–37.

Ferrara PJ. Expanding autonomy of the elderly in home health care programs. *New England Law Review.* 1990;25:421–455.

Guidelines for the medical management of the home-care patient. American Medical Association Home Care Advisory Panel. *Arch Fam Med.* 1993;2:194–206. Comments.

Hansell DA. AIDS and surrogate decision making. *Mt Sinai J Med.* 1991;58:375–378.

Hogstel MO, Gaul AL. Safety or autonomy. An ethical issue for clinical gerontological nurses. *J Gerontol Nurs.* 1991;17:6–11.

Howe EG. Attributing preferences and violating neutrality. *J Clin Ethics.* 1992;3:171–175. Comment.

Igoe S, Cascella S, Stockdale K. Ethics in the OR: DNR and patient autonomy. *Nurs Manage.* 1993;24:112A.

Kane RA, Caplan AL. *Ethical Conflicts in the Management of Home Care: The Case Manager's Dilemma.* New York, NY: Springer Publishing Co, Inc; 1993.

Kane RL, Kane RA. The impact of long-term-care financing on personal autonomy. *Generations.* 1990;14:86–89.

Kapp MB. *Geriatrics and the Law: Patient Rights and Professional Responsibilities.* 2nd ed. New York, NY: Springer Publishing Co, Inc; 1992.

Kimaid Y, Votava KM, Myers E. Patient advocacy: one agency's positive results with the administrative law judge process. *Home Healthcare Nurse.* 1994;12:29–32.

Kristoff B, Sellin S, Miller MP. Patients' rights and ethical dilemmas in home care: incorporation of psychological concepts. *Home Healthcare Nurse.* 1994;12:45–50. Published erratum appears in *Home Healthcare Nurse;* 1994;12:8.

Leibson CM. The role of the courts in terminating life-sustaining medical treatment. *Issues Law Med.* 1995;10:437–451.

Levenson JL, Pettrey L. Controversial decisions regarding treatment and DNR: an algorithmic Guide for the Uncertain in Decision-Making Ethics (GUIDE). *Am J Crit Care.* 1994;3:87–91.

Liaschenko J. The moral geography of home care. *ANS.* 1994;17:16–26.

Luce JM. Physicians do not have a responsibility to provide futile or unreasonable care if a patient or family insists. *Crit Care Med.* 1995;23:760–766. Comments.

Lynn J. Ethical issues in caring for elderly residents of nursing homes. *Prim Care.* 1986;13:295–306.

MacMillan-Scattergood D. Ethical conflicts in a prospective payment home health environment. *Nurs Economics.* 1986;4:165–170.

McClung JA. Time and language in bioethics: when patient and proxy appear to disagree. *J Clin Ethics.* 1995;6:39–43. Comments.

Meier DE, Cassel CK. Nursing home placement and the demented patient: a case presentation and ethical analysis. *Ann Intern Med.* 1986;1:98–105.

Milholland DK. Privacy and confidentiality of patient information. Challenges for nursing. *J Nurs Adm.* 1994;24:19–24.

Mullens A. The Dutch experience with euthanasia: lessons for Canada? *Can Med Assoc J.* 1995;152:1845–1852.

Olson E, Chichin E, Meyers H, Schulman E, Brennan F. Early experiences of an ethics consult team. *J Am Geriatr Soc.* 1994;42:437–441. Comments.

Osman H, Perlin TM. Patient self-determination and the artificial prolongation of life. *Health Soc Work.* 1994;19:245–252.

Outerbridge DE, Hersh AR. *Easing the Passage: A Guide for Prearranging and Ensuring a Pain-Free and Tranquil Death via a Living Will, Personal Medical Mandate, and Other Medical, Legal, and Ethical Resources.* New York, NY: HarperCollins; 1991.

Physicians and home health care. A report from the LSMS Physician/Patient Advocacy Committee. *J La State Med Soc.* 1994;146:269–271.

Post SG. Justice, community dialogue, and health care. *J Soc Philos.* 1992;23:23–34.

Power-Smith P, Evans M. Dementia. Communal confusion. *Nurs Times.* 1993;89:26–28.

Price DM. Forgoing treatment in an adult with no apparent treatment preferences: a case report. *Theor Med.* 1994;15:53–60.

Ruddick W. Transforming homes and hospitals. *Hastings Cent Rep.* 1994;24(suppl):S11–S14.

Sabatino CP. Client-rights regulations and the autonomy of home-care consumers. *Generations.* 1990;14:21–24.

Schwartz RL. Autonomy, futility, and the limits of medicine. *Camb Q Healthcare Ethics.* 1992;1:159–164.

Sprung CL, Eidelman LA, Steinberg A. Is the physician's duty to the individual patient or to society? *Crit Care Med.* 1995;23:618–620. Editorial; comment.

Stein PS. Are do-not-resuscitate, do-not-intubate orders appropriate for trauma patients? *AORN J.* 1993;58:576–577.

Turner JF, Mason T, Anderson D, Gulati A, Sbarbaro JA. Physicians' ethical responsibilities under co-pay insurance: should potential fiscal liability become part of informed consent? *J Clin Ethics*. 1995;6:68–72.

Van Bommel H. *Choices: For People Who Have a Terminal Illness, Their Families, and Their Caregivers*. Port Washington, NY: NC Press, 1986.

Weiler K, Helms LB, Buckwalter KC. A comparative study: guardianship petitions for adults and elder adults. *J Gerontol Nurs*. 1993;19:15–25.

Wenger NS, Halpern J. The physician's role in completing advance directives: ensuring patients' capacity to make healthcare decisions in advance. *J Clin Ethics*. 1994;5:320–323. Comments.

Williamson P, McCormick T, Taylor T. Who is the patient? A family case study of a recurrent dilemma in family practice. *J Fam Pract*. 1983;17:1039–1043.

Wilson-Barnett J. The nurse-patient relationship. In: Gillon R, ed. *Principles of Health Care Ethic*. Chicester, NY: John Wiley and Sons; 1994:367–376.

PATIENT CARE PLANNING

Agich GJ. Reassessing autonomy in long-term care. *Hastings Cent Rep*. 1990;20:12–17.

Agich GJ. *Autonomy and Long-Term Care*. New York, N.Y.: Oxford University Press; 1993.

Arras JD. The technological tether: an introduction to ethical and social issues in high-tech home care [and] executive summary of project conclusions. *Hastings Cent Rep*. 1994;24(suppl):S1–S3.

Bigler BR. Critical care nursing: expanding roles and responsibilities within the community. *Crit Care Nurs Clin North Am*. 1990;2:493–502.

Binstock RH. Long-term care for older people: moral and political challenges of access. In: Monagle JF, Thomasma DC, eds. *Health Care Ethics: Critical Issues*. Gaithersburg, MD: Aspen Publishers; 1994:158–167.

Bliss MR. Resources, the family and voluntary euthanasia. *Br J Gen Pract*. 1990;40(332):117–122.

Block JA. Evaluating the patient's capacity for making decisions. In: Dunkle RE, Wykle ML, eds. *Decision Making in Long-Term Care: Factors in Planning*. New York, NY: Springer Publishing Co, Inc; 1988:31–39.

Blumenfield S, Lowe JI. A template for analyzing ethical dilemmas in discharge planning. *Health Soc Work*. 1987;12:47–56.

Bovbjerg R, Held PJ, Diamond LH. Provider-patient relations and treatment choice in the era of fiscal incentives: the case of the End-Stage Renal Disease Program. *Milbank Q*. 1987;2:177–202.

Brock DW. Decisionmaking competence and risk. *Bioethics*. 1991;5:105–112.

Bromberg S, Cassel CK. Suicide in the elderly: the limits of paternalism. *J Am Geriatr Soc*. 1983;31:698–703.

Brummel-Smith K. Home health care: how long will it remain "low tech"? *Southern California Law Review*. 1991;65:491–502.

Callahan D. Families as caregivers: the limits of morality. *Arch Phys Med Rehabil*. 1988;69:323–328.

Cassel CK, Hays JR, Lynn J. Alzheimer's: decisions in terminal care. *Patient Care*. 1991;25(18):125–137.

Chadwick R, Russell J. Hospital discharge of frail elderly people: social and ethical considerations in the discharge decision-making process. *Ageing & Society*. 1989;9:277–295.

Cohen ES. The elderly mystique: impediment to advocacy and empowerment. *Generations*. 1990;14:13–16.

Collette J, Windt PY, Jahnigen DW. Medical decision-making, dying, and quality of life among the elderly. In: Smeeding TM, et al, eds. *Should Medical Care Be Rationed by Age?* Totowa, NJ: Rowman & Littlefield; 1987:99–118.

Collopy B, Dubler N, Zuckerman C. The ethics of home care: autonomy and accommodation. *Hastings Cent Rep*. 1990;20(2)(suppl):S1–S16.

Collopy BJ. Ethical dimensions of autonomy in long-term care. *Generations*. 1990;14:9–12.

Conflicts of interest: update on home care. In: *Code of Medical Ethics: Reports of the Council*. 5(1):Chicago, IL: American Medical Association; 1994:256–266. Report No. 58.

Dubler NN. Improving the discharge planning process: distinguishing between coercion and choice. *Gerontologist*. 1988;3(suppl):76–81.

Dubler NN. Autonomy and accommodation: mediating individual choice in the home setting. *Generations*. 1990;14:29–31.

Dubler NN. Individual advocacy as a governing principle. *J Case Manage*. 1992;1:82–86.

England M. Caregiver planning for a demented parent without crisis experience. *Sch Inq Nurs Pract*. 1994;8:295–313.

Esposito L. Home health case management: rural caregiving. *Home Healthcare Nurse*. 1994;12:38–43.

Estes CL. Cost containment and the elderly: conflict or challenge? *J Am Geriatr Soc*. 1988;1:65–72.

Feldman C, Olberding L, Shortridge L, Toole K, Zappin P. Decision making in case management of home healthcare clients. *J Nurs Adm.* 1993;23:33–38.

Ferrara PJ. Expanding autonomy of the elderly in home health care programs. *New England Law Review.* 1990;25:421–455.

Fox RC, Aiken LH, Messikomer CM. The culture of caring: AIDS and the nursing profession. *Milbank Q.* 1990; 68 (suppl):2:226–256.

Fry ST. Ethical issues in total parenteral nutrition. *Nutrition.* 1990;6:329–332.

Gartner MB, Twardon CA. Care guidelines: journey through the managed care maze. *J Wound Ostomy Continence Nurs.* 1995;22:118–121.

Gillick MR. *Choosing Medical Care in Old Age: What Kind, How Much, When to Stop.* Cambridge, Mass: Harvard University Press; 1994.

Haddad AM, Kapp MB. *Ethical and Legal Issues in Home Health Care: Case Studies and Analyses.* Norwalk, Conn: Appleton & Lange; 1991.

Havlir D, Brown L, Rousseau GK. Do not resuscitate discussions in a hospital-based home care program. *J Am Geriatr Soc.* 1989;1:52–54.

Hofland BF. Autonomy in long term care: background issues and a programmatic response. *Gerontologist.* 1988;3(suppl):3–9.

Jennings B, Callahan D, Caplan AL. Ethical challenges of chronic illness. *Hastings Cent Rep.* 1988;18(1)(suppl):S1–S16.

Kane RA, Caplan AL. *Ethical Conflicts in the Management of Home Care: The Case Manager's Dilemma.* New York, NY: Springer Publishing Co, Inc; 1993.

Kane RL, Kane RA. The impact of long-term-care financing on personal autonomy. *Generations.* 1990;14:86–89.

Kanoti GA. Writing a proposal for determining patient decisional capacity. *HEC Forum.* 1994;6:12–17.

Kapp MB. Are risk management and health care ethics compatible? *Perspect Healthcare Risk Manage.* 1991;11:2–7.

Kapp MB. *Geriatrics and the Law: Patient Rights and Professional Responsibilities.* 2nd ed. New York, NY: Springer Publishing Co, Inc; 1992.

Kapp MB. Who's the parent here? The family's impact on the autonomy of older persons. *Emory Law Journal.* 1992;41:773–803.

Kaufman J. Case management services for children with special health care needs. A family-centered approach. *J Case Manage.* 1992;1:53–56.

Keffer MJ, Keffer HL. U.S. ethics committees: perceived versus actual roles. *HEC Forum.* 1991;3(4):227–230.

Kerschner PA. Assuring access to long-term care: legal, ethical, and other barriers. In: Kapp MB, Pies HE, Doudera A, eds. *Legal and Ethical Care Aspects of Health Care for the Elderly.* Ann Arbor, MI: Health Administration Press; 1986:24–36.

Koop CE. Families caring for disabled need long-term support. *Health Progress.* 1986;67:52–54.

Lynn J. Ethical issues in caring for elderly residents of nursing homes. *Prim Care.* 1986;13:295–306.

Markson LJ, Steel K. Using advance directives in the home-care setting. *Generations.* 1990;14:25–28.

Meier B. Doctors' investments in home care grow, raising fears of ethical swamp. *New York Times;* 1993:A14. News.

Meier DE, Cassel CK. Nursing home placement and the demented patient: a case presentation and ethical analysis. *Ann Intern Med.* 1986;1:98–105.

Murphy DJ. Improving advance directives for healthy older people. *J Am Geriatr Soc.* 1990;38:1251–1256.

Orlowski JP. The HEC and conflicts of interest in the health care environment. *HEC Forum.* 1994;6:3–11.

Post S. An ethical perspective on caregiving in the family. *J Med Humanities Bioethics.* 1988;1:6–16.

Post SG. Justice, community dialogue, and health care. *J Soc Philos.* 1992;23:23–34.

Reisner A. Instructions for the Valley of the Shadow: a medical directive (living will). *United Synagogue Review.* 1992;44:22–23.

Riley PA, Fortinsky RH, Coburn AF. Developing consumer-centered quality assurance strategies for home care. A case management model. *J Case Manage.* 1992;1:39–48.

Rozell BR, Newman KL. Extending a critical path for patients who are ventilator dependent: nursing case management in the home setting. *Home Healthcare Nurse.* 1994;12:21–25.

Sabatino CP. Client-rights regulations and the autonomy of home-care consumers. *Generations.* 1990;14:21–24.

Schiedermayer D. *Putting the Soul Back in Medicine: Reflections on Compassion and Ethics.* Grand Rapids, Mich: Baker Books; 1994.

Scitovsky AA, Capron AM. Medical care at the end of life: the interaction of economics and ethics. In: Breslow L, Fielding JE, Lave LB, eds. *Annual Review of Public Health.* Palo Alto, CA: Annual Reviews; 1994:75.

Stoltzfus DP, Stamatos JM. An appraisal of the ethical issues involved in high-technology cancer pain relief. *J Clin Ethics*. 1991;2:113–115. Commentary.

Thomasma DC. Advance directives and health care for the elderly. In: Hackler C, Moseley R, Vawter DE, eds. *Advance Directives in Medicine*. New York: Praeger Publishers; 1989:93–109.

Waymack MH, Taler GA. *Medical Ethics and the Elderly: A Case Book*. Chicago, Ill: Pluribus Press, Inc; 1988.

Whiting M. Issues in community care. In: Brykczynska GM, ed. *Ethics in Paediatric Nursing*. London: Chapman and Hall; 1989:65–80.

Wicclair MR. *Ethics and the Elderly*. New York, NY: Oxford University Press; 1993.

Williamson P, McCormick T, Taylor T. Who is the patient? A family case study of a recurrent dilemma in family practice. *J Fam Pract*. 1983;17:1039–1043.

Wilson-Barnett J. The nurse-patient relationship. In: Gillon R, ed. *Principles of Health Care Ethics*. New York, NY: Wiley; 1994:367–376.

Young A, Pignatello CH, Taylor MB. Who's the boss? Ethical conflicts in home care. *Health Progress*. 1988;11:59–62.

Young PA. Home care characteristics that shape the exercise of autonomy: a view from the trenches. *Generations*. 1990;14:17–20.

Young PA, Pelaez M. The in-service education program of the Home Health Assembly of New Jersey. *Generations*. 1990;14:37–38.

PRACTICE GUIDELINES

American Nurses Association. Compendium of position statements on the nurse's role in end-of-life decisions. American Nurses Association Center for Ethics and Human Rights Task Force on the nurse's role in end-of-life decisions. American Nurses Association; 1992:1–13.

American Nurses Association position statement on nursing care and do-not-resuscitate decisions. *Ky Nurse*. 1993;41:16–17.

Barr P, Pinch WJ, Boardman K. Focus on ethics: ANA issues position statements. *Nebr Nurse*. 1993;26:21–22.

Conflicts of interest: update on home care. In: *Code of Medical Ethics: Reports of the Council*. 5(1). American Medical Association; 1994:266. Report No. 58.

Guidelines for the medical management of the home-care patient. American Medical Association Home Care Advisory Panel. *Arch Fam Med*. 1993;2:194–206. Comments.

Hudson T. Are futile-care policies the answer? Providers struggle with decisions for patients near the end of life. *Hosp Health Network.* 1994;68:26–30.

Jecker NS, Schneiderman LJ. An ethical analysis of the use of "futility" in the 1992 American Heart Association Guidelines for cardiopulmonary resuscitation and emergency cardiac care. *Arch Intern Med.* 1993;153:2195–2198. Comments.

Report of the Board of Trustees of the American Medical Association. Euthanasia/physician-assisted suicide: lessons in the Dutch experience. *Issues Law Med.* 1994;10:81–90.

Teno JM, Murphy D, Lynn J, Tosteson A, Desbiens N, Connors AF Jr, et al. Prognosis-based futility guidelines: does anyone win? SUPPORT Investigators. Study to Understand Prognoses and Preferences for Outcomes and Risks of Treatment. *J Am Geriatr Soc.* 1994;42:1202–1207.

PROFESSIONAL RELATIONS—PATIENT RELATIONS

Abel E. Ethics committees in home health agencies. *Public Health Nurs.* 1990;7:256–259.

Agich GJ. Reassessing autonomy in long-term care. *Hastings Cent Rep.* 1990;20:12–17.

Agich GJ. *Autonomy and Long-Term Care.* New York, NY: Oxford University Press; 1993.

Ahronheim J, Weber D. *Final Passages: Positive Choices for the Dying and Their Loved Ones.* New York, NY: Simon & Schuster; 1992.

Aroskar MA. Community health nurses: their most significant decision-making problems. *Nurs Clin North Am.* 1989;24:967–975.

Arras JD, Dubler NN. Bringing the hospital home. Ethical and social implications of high-tech home care. *Hastings Cent Rep.* 1994;24(suppl):S19–S28.

Asch DA, Hansen-Flaschen J, Lanken PN. Decisions to limit or continue life-sustaining treatment by critical care physicians in the United States: conflicts between physicians' practices and patients' wishes. *Am J Respir Crit Care Med.* 1995;151(pt 1):288–292. Comments.

Battin MP. Should we copy the Dutch? The Netherlands' practice of voluntary active euthanasia as a model for the United States. In: Misbin RI, ed. *Euthanasia: The Good of the Patient, the Good of Society.* Frederick, MD: University Publishing Group; 1992:95–103.

Bigler BR. Critical care nursing: expanding roles and responsibilities within the community. *Crit Care Nurs Clin North Am.* 1990;2:493–502.

Blumenfield S, Lowe JI. A template for analyzing ethical dilemmas in discharge planning. *Health Soc Work.* 1987;12:47–56.

Bovbjerg R, Held PJ, Diamond LH. Provider-patient relations and treatment choice in the era of fiscal incentives: the case of the End-Stage Renal Disease Program. *Milbank Q.* 1987;2:177–202.

Brown LM, Rousseau GK. Resuscitation status begins at home. *Am J Nurs.* 1990;4:24–26.

Burger AM, Erlen JA, Tesone L. Factors influencing ethical decision making in the home setting. *Home Healthcare Nurse.* 1992;10:16–20.

Cassel CK. Ethical issues in the conduct of research in long term care. *Gerontologist.* 1988;3(suppl):90–96.

Caswell D, Cryer HG. Case study: when the nurse and physician don't agree. *J Cardiovasc Nurs.* 1995;9:30–42.

Cohen CA, Meslin EM, Shulman KI. Dementia at home: ethical issues and clinical realities. In: Berg JM, Karlinsky H, Lowy FH, eds. *Alzheimer's Disease Research: Ethical Legal Issues.* Toronto: Cadwell; 1991:317–330.

Coll PP, Anderson D. Advanced directives for homebound patients. *J Am Board Fam Pract.* 1992;5:359–360. Letter; comment.

Collette J, Windt PY, Jahnigen DW. Medical decision-making, dying, and quality of life among the elderly. In: Smeeding TM, et al, eds. *Should Medical Care Be Rationed by Age?* Totowa, NJ: Rowman & Littlefield; 1987:49–118.

Collopy BJ. Ethical dimensions of autonomy in long-term care. *Generations.* 1990;14:9–12.

Curtis JR, Park DR, Krone MR, Pearlman RA. Use of the medical futility rationale in do-not-attempt-resuscitation orders. *JAMA.* 1995;273:124–128. Comments.

Dubler NN. Autonomy and accommodation: mediating individual choice in the home setting. *Generations.* 1990;14:29–31.

Dubler NN. Individual advocacy as a governing principle. *J Case Manage.* 1992;1:82–86.

Edwards BS. When the physician won't give up. *Am J Nurs.* 1993;93:34–37.

Report of the Board of Trustees of the American Medical Association. Euthanasia/physician-assisted suicide: lessons in the Dutch experience. *Issues Law Med.* 1994;1:81–90. Report.

Fins J. Encountering diversity: medical ethics and pluralism. *Journal of Religion & Health.* 1994;33:23–27.

Forrow L, Arnold RM, Parker LS. Preventive ethics: expanding the horizons of clinical ethics. *J Clin Ethics.* 1993;4:287–294. Comments.

Fox RC, Aiken LH, Messikomer CM. The culture of caring: AIDS and the nursing profession. *Milbank Q.* 1990;68 (suppl):2:226–256.

Guidelines for the medical management of the home-care patient. American Medical Association Home Care Advisory Panel. *Arch Fam Med.* 1993;2:194–206. Comments.

Haddad AM, Kapp MB. *Ethical and Legal Issues in Home Health Care: Case Studies and Analyses.* Norwalk, Conn: Appleton & Lange; 1991.

Hargrove MD Jr. A five-step approach to settling a dispute over futile care. *J La State Med Soc.* 1994;146:439–440.

Hiltunen EF, Puopolo AL, Marks GK, Marsden C, Kennard MJ, Follen MA, et al. The nurse's role in end-of-life treatment discussions: preliminary report from the SUPPORT Project. *J Cardiovasc Nurs.* 1995;9:68–77. Review.

Hofland BF. Autonomy in long term care: background issues and a programmatic response. *Gerontologist.* 1988;3(suppl):3–9.

Hudson T. Advance directives: still problematic for providers. *Hosp Health Network.* 1994;68:46.

Jennings B, Callahan D, Caplan AL. Ethical challenges of chronic illness. *Hastings Cent Rep.* 1988;1(suppl):S1–S16.

Johnson JE. Nurses vs doctors: the battle between the caregivers in health care reform. *Nursing Connections.* 1994;7:1–3.

Kane RA, Caplan AL. *Ethical Conflicts in the Management of Home Care: The Case Manager's Dilemma.* New York, NY: Springer Publishing Co, Inc; 1993.

Kapp MB. Who's the parent here? The family's impact on the autonomy of older persons. *Emory Law Journal.* 1992;41:773–803.

Kellogg FR, Crain M, Corwin J, Brickner PW. Life-sustaining interventions in frail elderly persons. Talking about choices. *Arch Intern Med.* 1992;152:2317–2320.

Kopelman LM. Conceptual and moral disputes about futile and useful treatments. *J Med Philos.* 1995;20:109–121.

Loewy EH. Suffering as a consideration in ethical decision making. *Camb Q Healthcare Ethics.* 1992;1:135–142.

MacDonald D. Unlimited claims on limited resources: entropy, health care, and a hospice world view. Third in a series. *Am J Hosp Palliat Care.* 1991;8:27–34.

MacLean DS, Wanzer SH. The physician's responsibility toward hopelessly ill patients. *N Engl J Med.* 1989;14:975–978. Letters and response.

Maher PL. Not safe at home: risk versus safety in home care. In: White GB, ed. *Ethical Dilemmas in Contemporary Nursing Practice.* Washington, DC: American Nurses Publishing; 1992.

Markson LJ, Steel K. Using advance directives in the home-care setting. *Generations.* 1990;14:25–28.

Markson LJ, Fanale J, Steel K, Kern D, Annas G. Implementing advance directives in the primary care setting. *Arch Intern Med.* 1994;154:2321–2327. Comments.

McEwen M. Promoting interdisciplinary collaboration. *Nurs Health Care.* 1994;15:304–307.

McWilliam CL, Brown JB, Carmichael JL, Lehman JM. A new perspective on threatened autonomy in elderly persons: the disempowering process. *Soc Sci Med.* 1994;38:327–338.

Paris NM, Hines J. Payer and provider relationships: the key to reshaping health care delivery. *Nurs Adm Q.* 1995;19:13–17.

Schiedermayer D. *Putting the Soul Back in Medicine: Reflections on Compassion and Ethics.* Grand Rapids, Mich: Baker Books; 1994.

Schneiderman LJ, Kaplan RM, Pearlman RA, Teetzel H. Do physicians' own preferences for life-sustaining treatment influence their perceptions of patients' preferences? *J Clin Ethics.* 1993;4:28–33.

Shaw AB. Acts of commission, omission, and demission or pulling the plug. *J R Soc Med.* 1995;88:18–19.

Sprung CL, Eidelman LA, Steinberg A. Is the physician's duty to the individual patient or to society? *Crit Care Med.* 1995;23:618–620. Editorial; comment.

Taylor EJ, Ferrell BR, Grant M, Cheyney L. Managing cancer pain at home: the decisional and ethical conflicts of patients, family caregivers, and homecare nurses. *Oncol Nurs Forum.* 1993;20:919–927.

Teres D. Trends from the United States with end of life decisions in the intensive care unit. *Intensive Care Med.* 1993;19:316–322. Review.

Thomasma DC. Models of the doctor-patient relationship and the ethics committee: part two. *Camb Q Healthcare Ethics.* 1994;3:10–26.

Traynor M. The views and values of community nurses and their managers: research in progress—one person's pain, another person's vision. *J Adv Nurs.* 1994;20:101–109.

Turner JF, Mason T, Anderson D, Gulati A, Sbarbaro JA. Physicians' ethical responsibilities under co-pay insurance: should potential fiscal liability become part of informed consent? *J Clin Ethics.* 1995;6:68–72.

Van Bommel H. *Choices: For People Who Have a Terminal Illness, Their Families, and Their Caregivers.* Port Washington, NY: NC Press; 1986.

Ventres W, Nichter M, Reed R, Frankel R. Limitation of medical care: an ethnographic analysis. *J Clin Ethics.* 1993;4:134–145. Comments.

Waisel DB, Truog RD. The cardiopulmonary resuscitation-not-indicated order: futility revisited. *Ann Intern Med.* 1995;122:304–308.

Waymack MH, Taler GA. *Medical Ethics and the Elderly: A Case Book.* Chicago, IL: Pluribus Press, Inc; 1988.

Wenger NS, Halpern J. The physician's role in completing advance directives: ensuring patients' capacity to make healthcare decisions in advance. *J Clin Ethics.* 1994;5:320–323. Comments.

Williamson P, McCormick T, Taylor T. Who is the patient? A family case study of a recurrent dilemma in family practice. *J Fam Pract.* 1983;17:1039–1043.

Wilson-Barnett J. The nurse-patient relationship. In: Gillon R, ed. *Principles of Health Care Ethics.* New York, NY: Wiley; 1994:367–376.

Young PA. Home care characteristics that shape the exercise of autonomy: a view from the trenches. *Generations.* 1990;14:17–20.

RESUSCITATION

Adams JG, Arnold R, Siminoff L, Wolfson AB. Ethical conflicts in the prehospital setting. *Ann Emerg Med.* 1992;21:1259–1265.

Adams JG, Derse AR, Gotthold WE, Mitchell JM, Moskop JC, Sanders AB. Ethical aspects of resuscitation. *Ann Emerg Med.* 1992;21:1273–1276.

Alpers A, Lo B. When is CPR futile? *JAMA.* 1995;273:156–158. Editorial; comment.

American Nurses Association. Compendium of position statements on the nurse's role in end-of-life decisions. American Nurses Association Center for Ethics and Human Rights Task Force on the nurse's role in end-of-life decisions. American Nurses Association; 1992:1–13.

American Nurses Association position statement on nursing care and do-not-resuscitate decisions. *Ky Nurse.* 1993;41:16–17.

Anderson B, Hall B. Parents' perceptions of decision making for children. *J Law Med Ethics*. 1995;23:15–19.

Barr P, Pinch WJ, Boardman K. Focus on ethics: ANA issues position statements. *Nebr Nurse*. 1993;26:21–22.

Baskett PJ. Ethics in cardiopulmonary resuscitation. *Resuscitation*. 1993;25:1–8. Editorial.

Bigler BR. Critical care nursing: expanding roles and responsibilities within the community. *Crit Care Nurs Clin North Am*. 1990;2:493–502.

Bliss MR. Resources, the family and voluntary euthanasia. *Br J Gen Pract*. 1990;40(332):117–122.

Brody BA, Halevy A. Is futility a futile concept? *J Med Philos*. 1995;20:123–144.

Brown LM, Rousseau GK. Resuscitation status begins at home. *Am J Nurs*. 1990;4:24–26.

Clark GD, Lucas K, Stephens L. Ethical dilemmas and decisions concerning the do-not-resuscitate patient undergoing anesthesia. *AANA J*. 1994;62:253–256.

Coll PP, Anderson D. Advanced directives for homebound patients. *J Am Board Fam Pract*. 1992;5:359–360. Letter; comment.

Curtis LL. DNR in the OR: ethical concerns and hospital policies. *Nurs Manage*. 1994;25:29–31.

Curtis JR, Park DR, Krone MR, Pearlman RA. Use of the medical futility rationale in do-not-attempt-resuscitation orders. *JAMA*. 1995;273:124–128. Comments.

Do-Not-Resuscitate (DNR) Decisions in the Context of Hospice Care. Arlington, Va: National Hospice Organization; 1992.

Dorff EN. "A time to be born and a time to die": a Jewish medical directive for health care. *United Synagogue Review*. 1992;45:20–22.

Ebell MH. When everything is too much. Quantitative approaches to the issue of futility. *Arch Fam Med*. 1995;4:352–356. Comments.

Edwards BS. When the physician won't give up. *Am J Nurs*. 1993;93:34–37.

Edwards BS. When the family can't let go. *Am J Nurs*. 1994;94:52–56.

Ethical considerations in resuscitation. *JAMA*. 1992;16:2282–2288.

Ethical issues of resuscitation. American College of Emergency Physicians. *Ann Emerg Med*. 1992;21:1277.

Finfer S, Theaker N, Raper R, Fisher M. The Hippocratic oath updated. Surrogates' decisions in resuscitation are of limited value. *BMJ*. 1994;309:953. Letter.

Garson KB. Do not resuscitate options in home care. *Home Healthcare Nurse.* 1992;10:21–23.

Guidelines for cardiopulmonary resuscitation and emergency cardiac care. Emergency Cardiac Care Committee and Subcommittees, American Heart Association. Part VIII. Ethical considerations in resuscitation. *JAMA.* 1992;16:2282–2288. Comments.

Havlir D, Brown L, Rousseau GK. Do not resuscitate discussions in a hospital-based home care program. *J Am Geriatr Soc.* 1989;1:52–54.

Hiltunen EF, Puopolo AL, Marks GK, Marsden C, Kennard MJ, Follen MA, et al. The nurse's role in end-of-life treatment discussions: preliminary report from the SUPPORT Project. *J Cardiovasc Nurs.* 1995;9:68–77. Review.

Hodgson PK. Dying at home. A review of the do-not-resuscitate process. *N C Med J.* 1995;56:97–99.

Igoe S, Cascella S, Stockdale K. Ethics in the OR: DNR and patient autonomy. *Nurs Manage.* 1993;24:112A.

Iserson KV, Rouse F. Prehospital DNR orders. *Hastings Cent Rep.* 1989;19:17–19. Case study and commentaries.

Iserson KV. Foregoing prehospital care: should ambulance staff always resuscitate? *J Med Ethics.* 1991;17:19–24.

Iserson KV. The "no code" tattoo—an ethical dilemma. *West J Med.* 1992;156:309–312.

Jecker NS, Schneiderman LJ. Ceasing futile resuscitation in the field: ethical considerations. *Arch Intern Med.* 1992;152:2392–2397. Review; comments.

Jecker NS, Schneiderman LJ. An ethical analysis of the use of "futility" in the 1992 American Heart Association Guidelines for cardiopulmonary resuscitation and emergency cardiac care. *Arch Intern Med.* 1993;153:2195–2198. Comments.

Jecker NS, Schneiderman LJ. Medical futility: the duty not to treat. *Camb Q Healthcare Ethics.* 1993;2:151–159.

Kapp MB. *Geriatrics and the Law: Patient Rights and Professional Responsibilities.* 2nd ed. New York, NY: Springer Publishing Co, Inc; 1992.

Koenig KL, Haynes B. Prehospital "do-not-resuscitate" orders—a new option. *West J Med.* 1993;159:602–603.

Levenson JL, Pettrey L. Controversial decisions regarding treatment and DNR: an algorithmic Guide for the Uncertain in Decision-Making Ethics (GUIDE). *Am J Crit Care.* 1994;3:87–91.

MacLean DS, Wanzer SH. The physician's responsibility toward hopelessly ill patients. *N Engl J Med*. 1989;14:975–978. Letters and response.

Marsden AK, Ng GA, Dalziel K, Cobbe SM. When is it futile for ambulance personnel to initiate cardiopulmonary resuscitation? *BMJ*. 1995;311:49–51.

Miles SH. Advanced directives to limit treatment: the need for portability. *J Am Geriatr Soc*. 1987;1:74–76. Editorial.

Muller JH. Shades of blue: the negotiation of limited codes by medical residents. *Soc Sci Med*. 1992;34:885–898.

Muller JH, Desmond B. Ethical dilemmas in a cross-cultural context. A Chinese example. *West J Med*. 1992;157:323–327.

Murakami JF, Wong WF. The decision to withdraw tube feeding. *Hawaii Med J*. 1995;54:485–489.

Murphy DJ. Improving advance directives for healthy older people. *J Am Geriatr Soc*. 1990;38:1251–1256.

Orlowski JP, Collins RL, Cancian SN. Forgoing life-supporting or death-prolonging therapy: a policy statement. *Cleve Clin J Med*. 1993;60:81–85.

Osman H, Perlin TM. Patient self-determination and the artificial prolongation of life. *Health Soc Work*. 1994;19:245–252.

Outerbridge DE, Hersh AR. *Easing the Passage: A Guide for Prearranging and Ensuring a Pain-Free and Tranquil Death via a Living Will, Personal Medical Mandate, and Other Medical, Legal, and Ethical Resources*. New York, NY: HarperCollins; 1991.

Price DM. Forgoing treatment in an adult with no apparent treatment preferences: a case report. *Theor Med*. 1994;15:53–60.

Reisner A. Instructions for the Valley of the Shadow: a medical directive (living will). *United Synagogue Review*. 1992;44:22–23.

Richard MS, Lassauniere JM. The role of a mobile palliative care team in the field of clinical ethics. *J Palliat Care*. 1992;8:36–39.

Robbins DA. Update: the removal of life supports in long-term care facilities. *J Long Term Care Adm*. 1985;13:3–5.

Robertson GS. Resuscitation and senility: a study of patients' opinions. *J Med Ethics*. 1993;19:104–107. Comments.

Rusin MJ. Communicating with families of rehabilitation patients about "do not resuscitate" decisions. *Arch Phys Med Rehabil*. 1992;73:922–925.

Schiedermayer D. *Putting the Soul Back in Medicine: Reflections on Compassion and Ethics*. Grand Rapids, Mich: Baker Books; 1994.

Singer PA, Cohen R, Robb A, Rothman A. The ethics objective structured clinical examination. *J Gen Intern Med.* 1993;8:23–28. Comments.

Singer PA, Robb A, Cohen R, Norman G, Turnbull J. Evaluation of a multicenter ethics objective structured clinical examination. *J Gen Intern Med.* 1994;9:690–692. Comments.

Smith ML. Futile medical treatment and patient consent. *Cleve Clin J Med.* 1993;60:151–154. Review.

Stein PS. Are do-not-resuscitate, do-not-intubate orders appropriate for trauma patients? *AORN J.* 1993;58:576–577.

Taylor RM, Lantos JD. The politics of medical futility. *Issues Law Med.* 1995;11:3–12.

Teres D. Trends from the United States with end of life decisions in the intensive care unit. *Intensive Care Med.* 1993;19:316–322. Review.

Terry M, Zweig S. Prevalence of advance directives and do-not-resuscitate orders in community nursing facilities. *Arch Fam Med.* 1994;3:141–145.

Thomasma DC. Models of the doctor-patient relationship and the ethics committee: part two. *Camb Q Healthcare Ethics.* 1994;3:10–26.

Van Bommel H. *Choices: For People Who Have a Terminal Illness, Their Families, and Their Caregivers.* Port Washington, NY: NC Press; 1986.

Ventres W, Nichter M, Reed R, Frankel R. Limitation of medical care: an ethnographic analysis. *J Clin Ethics.* 1993;4:134–145. Comments.

Waisel DB, Truog RD. The cardiopulmonary resuscitation-not-indicated order: futility revisited. *Ann Intern Med.* 1995;122:304–308.

Wanzer SH. The physician's responsibility toward hopelessly ill patients: a second look. *N Engl J Med.* 1989;320:844–849.

Waymack MH, Taler GA. *Medical Ethics and the Elderly: A Case Book.* Chicago, Ill: Pluribus Press, Inc; 1988.

Wicclair MR. *Ethics and the Elderly.* New York, NY: Oxford University Press; 1993.

TREATMENT REFUSAL

Adams JG, Derse AR, Gotthold WE, Mitchell JM, Moskop JC, Sanders AB. Ethical aspects of resuscitation. *Ann Emerg Med.* 1992;21:1273–1276.

Ahronheim J, Weber D. *Final Passages: Positive Choices for the Dying and Their Loved Ones.* New York, NY: Simon & Schuster, Inc; 1992.

Bigler BR. Critical care nursing: expanding roles and responsibilities within the community. *Crit Care Nurs Clin North Am.* 1990;2:493–502.

Bliss MR. Resources, the family and voluntary euthanasia. *Br J Gen Pract.* 1990;40(332):117–122.

Brock DW. Decisionmaking competence and risk. *Bioethics.* 1991;5:105–112.

Brummel-Smith K. Home health care: how long will it remain "low tech"? *Southern California Law Review.* 1991;65:491–502.

Coll PP, Anderson D. Advanced directives for homebound patients. *J Am Board Fam Pract.* 1992;5:359–360. Letter; comment.

Collopy B, Dubler N, Zuckerman C. The ethics of home care: autonomy and accommodation. *Hastings Cent Rep.* 1990;20(2)(suppl):S1–S16.

Collopy BJ. Ethical dimensions of autonomy in long-term care. *Generations.* 1990;14:9–12.

Cranford RE. The role of the ethics consultant in personal ethical dilemmas. In: Culver CM, ed. *Ethics at the Bedside.* Hanover, NH: University Press of New England; 1990:194–206.

Cummings NB. Social ethical, and legal issues involved in chronic maintenance dialysis. In: Maher JF, ed. *Replacement of Renal Function by Dialysis: A Textbook of Dialysis.* 3rd ed. Boston: Kluwer Acad; 1989:1141–1158.

Do-Not-Resuscitate (DNR) Decisions in the Context of Hospice Care. Arlington, Va: National Hospice Organization; 1992.

Dorff EN. "A time to be born and a time to die": a Jewish medical directive for health care. *United Synagogue Review.* 1992;45:20–22.

Dubler NN. Improving the discharge planning process: distinguishing between coercion and choice. *Gerontologist.* 1988;3(suppl):76–81.

Ethical considerations in resuscitation. *JAMA.* 1992;16:2282–2288.

Gillick MR. *Choosing Medical Care in Old Age: What Kind, How Much, When to Stop.* Cambridge, Mass: Harvard University Press; 1994.

Herr SS, Bostrom BA, Barton RS. No place to go: refusal of life-sustaining treatment by competent persons with physical disabilities. *Issues Law Med.* 1992;8:3–36. Review.

Hogue EE. Child neglect in home care: weighing legal and ethical issues. *Pediatr Nurs.* 1993;19:496–498.

Iserson KV. Foregoing prehospital care: should ambulance staff always resuscitate? *J Med Ethics.* 1991;17:19–24.

Iserson KV, Rouse F. Prehospital DNR orders. *Hastings Cent Rep.* 1989;19:17–19. Case study and commentaries.

Kanoti GA. Writing a proposal for determining patient decisional capacity. *HEC Forum.* 1994;6:12–17.

Kapp MB. Are risk management and health care ethics compatible? *Persp Healthcare Risk Manage.* 1991;11:2–7.

Kapp MB. *Geriatrics and the Law: Patient Rights and Professional Responsibilities.* 2nd ed. New York, NY: Springer Publishing Co, Inc; 1992.

Key ethical issues in palliative care: evidence to House of Lords Select Committee on Medical Ethics. 1993. The Council, London, England.

MacLean DS, Wanzer SH. The physician's responsibility toward hopelessly ill patients. *N Engl J Med.* 1989;321(14):975–978. Letters and response.

Mahoney J, Singer PA, Lowy FH, Hilberman M, Mitchell A, Stroud CE, et al. Cost savings at the end of life. *N Engl J Med.* 1994;331:477–478. Letters and response.

Miles SH. Advanced directives to limit treatment: the need for portability. *J Am Geriatr Soc.* 1987;1:74–76. Editorial.

Outerbridge DE, Hersh AR. *Easing the Passage: A Guide for Prearranging and Ensuring a Pain-Free and Tranquil Death via a Living Will, Personal Medical Mandate, and Other Medical, Legal, and Ethical Resources.* New York, NY: HarperCollins; 1991.

Price DM. Forgoing treatment in an adult with no apparent treatment preferences: a case report. *Theor Med.* 1994;15:53–60.

Thomasma DC. Advance directives and health care for the elderly. In: Hackler C, Moseley R, Vawter DE, eds. *Advance Directives in Medicine.* New York, NY: Praeger Press; 1989:93–109.

Van Bommel H. *Choices: For People Who Have a Terminal Illness, Their Families, and Their Caregivers.* Port Washington, NY: NC Press; 1986.

Wanzer SH. The physician's responsibility toward hopelessly ill patients: a second look. *N Engl J Med.* 1989;320:844–849.

Wicclair MR. *Ethics and the Elderly.* New York, NY: Oxford University Press; 1993.

Young A, Pignatello CH, Taylor MB. Who's the boss? Ethical conflicts in home care. *Health Progress.* 1988;11:59–62.

Index

Note: Page numbers in *Italics* indicate material in figures, tables, or exhibits.

About the Author

Dennis A. Robbins, PhD, MPH, is a nationally recognized clinical ethics and health law consultant. He has lectured and offered programs in 46 states and abroad. He has served as director and chair of the Graduate Program in Health Services Administration, where he taught courses in health law, ethics, and health policy.

Dr. Robbins was a National Fund for Medical Education Fellow in the Kennedy Interfaculty Program in Medical Ethics through the Division of Legal Medicine at Harvard University's Schools of Public Health and Medicine. He studied law at Harvard and the University of Mississippi and has had three postdoctoral fellowships in medical ethics and health law. He has consulted extensively on policy development, ethics and managed care, withholding/withdrawing life prolonging medical procedures, ethics committees, conflict resolution, and hospice.

He worked as an ethics consultant for a large Massachusetts General Hospital–affiliated oncology service and served as the Director of Medical Ethics at Sinai Hospital in Detroit as well as a clinical ethicist for the Veterans Administration in various locations across the country. During his postdoctoral work at Harvard, he was an intern on a large oncology unit and co-coordinator of clinical ethics rounds at Children's Hospital in Boston.

Dr. Robbins has written over 150 articles and reviews and is the author of *Legal and Ethical Issues in Cancer in the United States* (1984) and *Ethical Dimensions of Clinical Medicine* (1982). He was also the medical ethics editor for the *Journal of Emergency Nursing* for four years.

Dr. Robbins has been an advisor to and offered seminars for such organizations as the American Medical Association, the American Board of Utilization Review and Quality Assurance Physicians, the American College of Health Care Executives, the Joint Commission on Accreditation of Healthcare Organizations, the American Hospital Association, the National Hospice Association, the American Health Care Association, and the American Association of Homes and Housing for the Aged, and to legislators, judges, policymakers, and government.

Dr. Robbins is an adjunct associate professor at the Chicago Medical School and teaches several courses in legal and ethical issues in managed care and health care reform at Loyola Strich School of Medicine. In addition, he is president of Integrated Decisions Ethics Alternatives and Solutions (IDEAS), an ethics and health law consulting firm he started ten years ago.